Alcoholic Liver Disease

Editor

STANLEY MARTIN COHEN

CLINICS IN
LIVER DISEASE

www.liver.theclinics.com

Consulting Editor
NORMAN GITLIN

August 2016 • Volume 20 • Number 3

ELSEVIER

1600 John F. Kennedy Boulevard ● Suite 1800 ● Philadelphia, Pennsylvania, 19103-2899

http://www.theclinics.com

CLINICS IN LIVER DISEASE Volume 20, Number 3
August 2016 ISSN 1089-3261, ISBN-13: 978-0-323-45973-0

Editor: Kerry Holland
Developmental Editor: Meredith Clinton

Clinics in Liver Disease (ISSN 1089-3261) is published quarterly by Elsevier Inc., 360 Park Avenue South, New York, NY 10010-1710. Months of issue are February, May, August, and November. Business and Editorial Offices: 1600 John F. Kennedy Blvd., Ste. 1800, Philadelphia, PA 19103-2899. Customer Service Office: 3251 Riverport Lane, Maryland Heights, MO 63043. Periodicals postage paid at New York, NY and additional mailing offices. Subscription prices are $275.00 per year (U.S. individuals), $100.00 per year (U.S. student/resident), $453.00 per year (U.S. institutions), $395.00 per year (international individuals), $200.00 per year (international student/resident), $562.00 per year (international instituitions), $340.00 per year (Canadian individuals), $200.00 per year (Canadian student/resident), and $562.00 per year (Canadian institutions). Foreign air speed delivery is included in all *Clinics* subscription prices. All prices are subject to change without notice. **POSTMASTER:** Send address changes to *Clinics in Liver Disease*, Elsevier Health Sciences Division, Subscription Customer Service, 3251 Riverport Lane, Maryland Heights, MO 63043. **Customer Service: Telephone: 1-800-654-2452 (U.S. and Canada); 314-447-8871 (outside U.S. and Canada). Fax: 314-447-8029. E-mail: journalscustomer service-usa@elsevier.com (for print support); journalsonlinesupport-usa@elsevier.com (for online support).**

Reprints. For copies of 100 or more of articles in this publication, please contact the Commercial Reprints Department, Elsevier Inc., 360 Park Avenue South, New York, NY 10010-1710. Tel.: 212-633-3874; Fax: 212-633-3820; E-mail: reprints@elsevier.com.

Clinics in Liver Disease is covered in *MEDLINE/PubMed (Index Medicus)*, Science Citation Index Expanded, Journal Citation Reports/Science Edition, and Current Contents/Clinical Medicine.

Contributors

CONSULTING EDITOR

NORMAN GITLIN, MD, FRCP (LONDON), FRCPE (EDINBURGH), FAASLD, FACP, FACG
Formerly, Professor of Medicine, Chief of Hepatology, Emory University; Currently, Consultant, Atlanta Gastroenterology Associates, Atlanta, Georgia

EDITOR

STANLEY MARTIN COHEN, MD, FAASLD, FACG
Medical Director, Hepatology, Digestive Health Institute, University Hospitals Case Medical Center; Professor of Medicine, Division of Gastroenterology and Liver Disease, Case Western Reserve University School of Medicine, Cleveland, Ohio

AUTHORS

JOSEPH AHN, MD, MS, FACG
Division of Gastroenterology, Department of Medicine, Oregon Health and Science University, Portland, Oregon

SANATH ALLAMPATI, MD
Department of Clinical Nutrition, Cleveland Clinic Foundation, Cleveland, Ohio

LINDSAY ALPERT, MD
Gastrointestinal and Hepatic Pathology Fellow, Department of Pathology, The University of Chicago, Chicago, Illinois

KRISTINA RACHEL CHACKO, MD
Division of Gastroenterology and Liver Diseases, Montefiore Medical Center, Bronx, New York

CHRISTINE CHAN, MD
Fellow, Division of Gastroenterology and Hepatology, Northwestern University Feinberg School of Medicine, Chicago, Illinois

MICHAEL R. CHARLTON, MD, FRCP
Professor of Medicine, Chief of Hepatology, Medical Director of Liver Transplantation, Intermountain Transplant Center, Intermountain Medical Center, Murray, Utah

RYAN E. CHILDERS, MD
Division of Gastroenterology, Department of Medicine, Oregon Health and Science University, Portland, Oregon

SRINIVASAN DASARATHY, MD
Departments of Gastroenterology, Hepatology and Pathobiology, Lerner Research Institute, Cleveland Clinic, Cleveland, Ohio

MOHANNAD F. DUGUM, MD
Division of Gastroenterology, Hepatology and Nutrition, University of Pittsburgh, Pittsburgh, Pennsylvania

WINSTON DUNN, MD
Associate Professor, Gastroenterology and Hepatology, The University of Kansas Medical Center, Kansas City, Kansas

JUAN F. GALLEGOS-OROZCO, MD
Assistant Professor of Medicine, Medical Director of Hepatology and Liver Transplantation, Division of Gastroenterology, Hepatology and Nutrition, University of Utah School of Medicine, Salt Lake City, Utah

PIERRE M. GHOLAM, MD
Case Western Reserve University School of Medicine; Liver Center of Excellence, Digestive Health Institute, University Hospitals Case Medical Center, Cleveland, Ohio

ROBERT GISH, MD
Division of Hepatology, St. Joseph's Hospital and Medical Center, Creighton University School of Medicine, Phoenix, Arizona; Division of Hepatology and Gastroenterology, Stanford University Hospitals and Clinics, Palo Alto, California

JOHN HART, MD
Professor, Department of Pathology, The University of Chicago, Chicago, Illinois

STEPHEN HOLT, MD, MS, FACP
Assistant Professor, Section of General Internal Medicine, Department of Medicine, Yale School of Medicine, New Haven, Connecticut

CHRISTINE C. HSU, MD
Assistant Professor of Clinical Medicine, University of Pennsylvania, Philadelphia, Pennsylvania

KARTIK JOSHI, MBS, BS
Division of Hepatology, St. Joseph's Hospital and Medical Center, Creighton University School of Medicine, Phoenix, Arizona

ANITA KOHLI, MD, MS
Divisions of Hepatology and Infectious Disease, St. Joseph's Hospital and Medical Center, Creighton University School of Medicine, Phoenix, Arizona

KRIS V. KOWDLEY, MD
Director of Liver Care Network and Organ Care Research, Swedish Liver Care Network, Swedish Medical Center, Seattle, Washington

JOSH LEVITSKY, MD, MS
Associate Professor of Medicine and Surgery; Program Director, Gastroenterology and Transplant Hepatology Fellowships, Division of Gastroenterology and Hepatology, Comprehensive Transplant Center, Northwestern University Feinberg School of Medicine; Director of Liver Research, Northwestern University, Chicago, Illinois

MICHAEL R. LUCEY, MD
Professor and Chief, Division of Gastroenterology and Hepatology, Department of Medicine, University of Wisconsin School of Medicine and Public Health, Madison, Wisconsin

RICHARD MANCH, MD
Division of Hepatology, St. Joseph's Hospital and Medical Center, Creighton University School of Medicine, Phoenix, Arizona

ARTHUR J. McCULLOUGH, MD
Department of Gastroenterology and Hepatology, Digestive Disease Institute, Cleveland Clinic, Cleveland, Ohio

KEVIN D. MULLEN, MD, FACP
Bioscientific Staff, MetroHealth Medical Center, Cleveland, Ohio

PAULINA K. PHILLIPS, MD
Gastroenterology Fellow, Division of Gastroenterology and Hepatology, Department of Medicine, University of Wisconsin School of Medicine and Public Health, Madison, Wisconsin

JOHN REINUS, MD
Medical Director of Liver Transplantation, Montefiore Medical Center, Bronx, New York; Professor of Clinical Medicine, Albert Einstein College of Medicine, New York, New York

VIJAY H. SHAH, MD
Professor of Medicine, Gastroenterology Research Unit, Division of Gastroenterology and Hepatology, Mayo Clinic, Rochester, Minnesota

JEANETTE TETRAULT, MD, FACP
Associate Professor, Section of General Internal Medicine, Department of Medicine, Yale School of Medicine, New Haven, Connecticut

Contents

> Liver disease from excessive alcohol consumption is an important cause of morbidity and mortality worldwide. There is a clear relationship between alcohol and a variety of health and socioeconomic problems. According to the World Health Organization, 3.3 million people die of alcohol-related causes annually. Despite public knowledge of its potential adverse effects, alcohol consumption and the morbidity and mortality from alcoholic liver disease (ALD) have increased. ALD comprises a spectrum of injury, including simple steatosis, acute alcoholic hepatitis, and cirrhosis. Rather than being distinct disease entities, these pathologic processes frequently overlap.

> Unhealthy alcohol use is common, and routine screening is essential to identify patients and initiate appropriate treatment. At-risk or hazardous drinking is best managed with brief interventions, which can be performed by any provider and are designed to enhance patients' motivations and promote behavioral change. Alcohol withdrawal can be managed, preferably with benzodiazepines, using a symptom-triggered approach. Twelve-step programs and provider-driven behavioral therapies have robust data supporting their effectiveness and patients with alcohol use disorder should be referred for these services. Research now support the use of several FDA-approved medications that aid in promoting abstinence and reducing heavy drinking.

> Alcoholic liver disease includes a broad clinical-histological spectrum from simple steatosis, cirrhosis, acute alcoholic hepatitis with or without cirrhosis to hepatocellular carcinoma as a complication of cirrhosis. The pathogenesis of alcoholic liver disease can be conceptually divided into (1) ethanol-mediated liver injury, (2) inflammatory immune response to injury, (3) intestinal permeability and microbiome changes. Corticosteroids may improve outcomes, but this is controversial and probably only impacts short-term survival. New pathophysiology-based therapies are under study, including antibiotics, caspase inhibition, interleukin-22, anakinra, FXR agonist and others. These studies provide hope for better future outcomes for this difficult disease.

therapy and it decreases mortality and morbidity significantly. Alcoholic cirrhosis can cause varices that need to be followed closely with upper endoscopy to prevent or treat hemorrhage. In this review, we describe an approach to long-term management of ALD.

In this review we critically assess the literature to evaluate the level of risk posed by alcohol as both a primary etiology of hepatocellular carcinoma (HCC) and as a cofactor in its development. Although there have been conflicting findings, based on the body of evidence to date, it appears that the linkage between compensated alcoholic liver disease-associated cirrhosis and HCC is best characterized as medium-high risk, with the risk increasing with age and with quantity and duration of alcohol consumption, and is more pronounced in females. While abstinence is the most effective way to reduce HCC risk, its effect seems largely dependent on the severity of liver damage at the point of cessation. Alcohol clearly interacts with other etiologies and conditions including viral hepatitis B and C, hereditary hemochromatosis, diabetes, and obesity to increase the risk for developing HCC, either synergistically or additively. Continued progress in genetics, especially through mechanistic-based and genome-wide association studies may ultimately identify which single nucleotide polymorphisms are risk factors for the onset of alcoholic liver disease and its progression to HCC and lead to the development of targeted therapeutics which may help providers better manage at-risk patients.

Alcohol consumption is often a comorbid condition in other chronic liver diseases. It has been shown to act in synergy to increase liver injury in viral hepatitis, hereditary hemochromatosis, and nonalcoholic fatty liver disease (NAFLD), leading to an increased risk of cirrhosis, hepatocellular carcinoma, and liver-related mortality. Data suggest that modest alcohol consumption may be inversely related to the risk of developing NAFLD and lower rates of progression of NAFLD to nonalcoholic steatohepatitis (NASH). This article reviews data on the relationship between alcohol consumption and other chronic liver diseases.

Acute and chronic alcohol use leads to an impaired immune response and dysregulated inflammatory state that contributes to a markedly increased risk of infection. Via shared mechanisms of immune-mediated injury, alcohol can alter the clinical course of viral infections such as hepatitis B, hepatitis C, and human immunodeficiency virus. These effects are most evident in patients with alcoholic hepatitis and cirrhosis. This article provides an overview of alcohol's effect on the immune system and contribution to the risks and outcomes of specific infectious diseases.

CLINICS IN LIVER DISEASE

THE CLINICS ARE AVAILABLE ONLINE!
Access your subscription at:
www.theclinics.com

Preface

Alcoholic Liver Disease

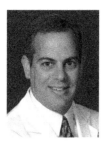

Stanley Martin Cohen, MD, FAASLD, FACG
Editor

Alcoholic liver disease (ALD) remains a major health issue with significant physical, psychological, and financial effects. The disease can present with a range of hepatic manifestations, including alcoholic fatty liver disease, acute alcoholic hepatitis (AH), and alcoholic cirrhosis. In this issue of *Clinics in Liver Disease*, it has been my privilege as Guest Editor to work with a distinguished group of authors to explore a wide range of topics on this subject.

Drs Chacko and Reinus set the stage for this issue with an overview of the spectrum of ALD. Recognizing at-risk drinking and alcoholism can be very difficult; Drs Holt and Tetrault give a comprehensive review on all aspects of unhealthy alcohol use. Drs Dunn and Shah then provide an excellent overview on the pathogenesis of ALD. Drs Childers and Ahn provide a thorough review on the diagnosis of ALD, with a focus on clinical aspects, lab parameters, and biopsy results. To further review the pathology and liver biopsy aspects of ALD, Drs Alpert and Hart provide a pathologist's perspective on ALD.

This issue then moves on to the clinical syndrome of AH. This topic is given a significant amount of articles due to its high mortality and significant clinical impact. Dr Gholam outlines the various prognostic scoring models utilized for AH. Drs Dugum and McCullough then provide a thorough review of the clinical aspects of AH. Given the high mortality associated with severe AH, Drs Phillips and Lucey provide us with an overview of the treatment options for AH. Then, Drs Gallegos-Orozco and Charlton cover the controversial topic of liver transplantation for ALD and AH.

Malnutrition can be considered one of the most frequent (and overlooked) complications associated with ALD. Dr Dasarathy provides a very thorough review of this topic.

As medical care improves and alcoholic patients live longer, we need an approach to caring for these patients. Drs Allampati and Mullen provide a review on the long-term management of patients with ALD. Advanced liver disease and cirrhosis account for the majority of cases of hepatocellular carcinoma (HCC) in the United States. However, there has been some debate about whether ALD is a significant predisposing risk

Clin Liver Dis 20 (2016) xiii–xiv
http://dx.doi.org/10.1016/j.cld.2016.05.001
1089-3261/16/$ – see front matter © 2016 Published by Elsevier Inc.

liver.theclinics.com

factor for HCC. Drs Joshi, Kohli, Manch, and Gish review this topic. While it is clear that alcohol can cause liver disease directly, there is less written on the effects of alcohol on other chronic liver diseases. Drs Hsu and Kowdley cover this subject with a focus on the effects of alcohol on patients with fatty liver disease, chronic viral hepatitis, and hemochromatosis. Finally, Drs Chan and Levitsky provide a review on the topic of infection in patients with ALD.

I wish to acknowledge many people in the production of this issue. I must thank Dr Norman Gitlin for asking me to serve as Guest Editor. I am also grateful to the expert panel of authors who have produced such amazing manuscripts. I would like to thank the publisher, and in particular, Meredith Clinton, without whose tireless work and support this issue may never have made it to press. And finally, I would like to thank my family: my son, Ben, and my lovely wife, Marianne. The considerable time that I spent on this journal was time away from them. Despite that, their support was always with me.

Stanley Martin Cohen, MD, FAASLD, FACG
Digestive Health Institute
University Hospitals Case Medical Center
Division of Gastroenterology and Liver Disease
Case Western Reserve
University School of Medicine
11100 Euclid Avenue
Cleveland, OH 44106-5066, USA

E-mail address:
Stanley.Cohen@UHhospitals.org

Spectrum of Alcoholic Liver Disease

Kristina Rachel Chacko, MD[a], John Reinus, MD[b],*

KEYWORDS

- Alcoholic liver disease • Epidemiology of alcohol abuse • Alcoholic hepatitis
- Risk factors for alcoholic liver disease

KEY POINTS

- Alcoholic liver disease is a major cause of socioeconomic and health problems in the developed world.
- The risk of alcoholic liver disease is affected by gender, age, genetics, drinking patterns, and obesity.
- The spectrum of alcoholic liver disease includes simple steatosis, acute alcoholic hepatitis, and alcoholic cirrhosis.

INTRODUCTION

Liver disease from excessive alcohol consumption is an important cause of morbidity and mortality worldwide. Fermented beverages were first made in the Neolithic era (10,000 BC), and subsequently, the relationship between alcohol and a variety of health and socioeconomic problems has become increasingly evident.[1] According to the World Health Organization (WHO), 3.3 million people die of alcohol-related causes annually.[2] Despite public knowledge of its potential adverse effects, alcohol consumption has increased and, with it, morbidity and mortality from alcoholic liver disease (ALD).[3] ALD comprises a spectrum of injury, including simple steatosis, acute alcoholic hepatitis, and cirrhosis. Rather than being distinct disease entities, these pathologic processes frequently overlap.

EPIDEMIOLOGY OF ALCOHOLIC LIVER DISEASE

ALD has been extensively studied for many years. However, an improved understanding of chronic viral hepatitis and nonalcoholic fatty liver disease has altered the interpretation of prior decades of epidemiologic data concerning the health effects of alcohol abuse. It is estimated that approximately 67.3% of the adult United States

Disclosure: The authors have nothing to disclose.
[a] Division of Gastroenterology & Liver Diseases, Montefiore Medical Center, Bronx, NY, USA;
[b] Department of Clinical Medicine, Albert Einstein College of Medicine, 111 East 210th Street, Rosenthal 2C, Bronx, NY 10467, USA
* Corresponding author.
E-mail address: jreinus@montefiore.org

population drinks alcohol and 7.4% meet criteria for alcohol abuse.[4] Globally, the WHO estimates that individuals older than age 15 years drink an average of 6.2 L of pure alcohol per year (**Fig. 1**); the equivalent of 13.5 g per day (**Table 1**). There is great regional variability in alcohol consumption caused by socioeconomic, cultural, and religious factors, with the highest levels in Europe and the Americas and the lowest levels in south-east Asia and eastern Mediterranean countries.[2] As a result, the burden of alcohol-related disease and disability is highest in the developed world. A small proportion of drinkers consume most of the alcohol imbibed; for example, in the United States, 20% of drinkers are responsible for 80% of alcohol consumption.[4] In 1998, estimated alcohol-related health-care costs in the United States were $26.5 billion, and in 2005 an estimated 1.152 million life-years were lost from premature mortality caused by alcohol-related disorders.[4,5]

Age and Alcoholic Liver Injury

People often start drinking alcohol at a young age, and, as a result, ALD may affect individuals of any age. Based on years of life lost because of premature mortality, ALD is most often seen in persons aged 45 to 54 years, followed by those aged 35 to 44 years.[5] Recently, there has been an increase in alcohol abuse among the elderly, with up to 10% to 15% of elderly primary-care patients meeting criteria for alcohol abuse; as a result, this subpopulation has experienced an increase in alcohol-related hospitalizations and deaths from alcoholic cirrhosis.[3,6]

Gender and Alcoholic Liver Injury

Men consume significantly more alcohol than women and consequently have 9 times more alcohol-related liver disease.[7] However, women are more vulnerable to the hepatotoxic effects of alcohol and, compared with men, have greater than twice the relative risk of ALD and cirrhosis for any given alcohol intake.[8] Women who consume 7 to 13 alcoholic beverages each week are at risk of developing ALD, compared with 14 to 27 for men. Female gender also is considered an independent risk factor for fibrosis progression in individuals with simple steatosis.[9]

Ethnicity, Genetics, and Alcoholic Liver Disease

The effect of ethnicity on the development and outcome of ALD is an important issue complicated by the changes in public reporting practices regarding race over time. Mortality data that distinguished between Hispanic and non-Hispanic white people showed that white Hispanic men had the highest death rates from cirrhosis (with mention of alcohol) followed by black non-Hispanic men, with Hispanic men of Mexican origin at highest risk.[10,11] Hispanic men also seem to develop ALD including alcoholic hepatitis and cirrhosis at a significantly younger age than do white non-Hispanic men.[12] American Indians and native Alaskans had a significantly higher mortality from chronic ALD compared with white people.[13]

Recently, genome-wide association studies found that the patatinlike phospholipase-domain containing protein 3 (PNPLA3) gene is associated with increased hepatic fat content and an increased risk of developing both alcoholic and nonalcoholic fatty liver disease.[14] A meta-analysis found that the PNPLA3 polymorphism increases the risk of developing the entire spectrum of ALD and is associated with increased disease severity.[15] The PNPLA3 polymorphism seems to be more prevalent in persons of native-American ancestry from South America compared with non-native South Americans; for example, those of Spanish, European, and African ancestry.[16] A high frequency of PNPLA3 variants and a strong association of these variants with increased serum alanine aminotransferase (ALT) levels has been found in indigenous Mexican and

Total alcohol per capita (15+ years) consumption, in litres of pure alcohol, 2010

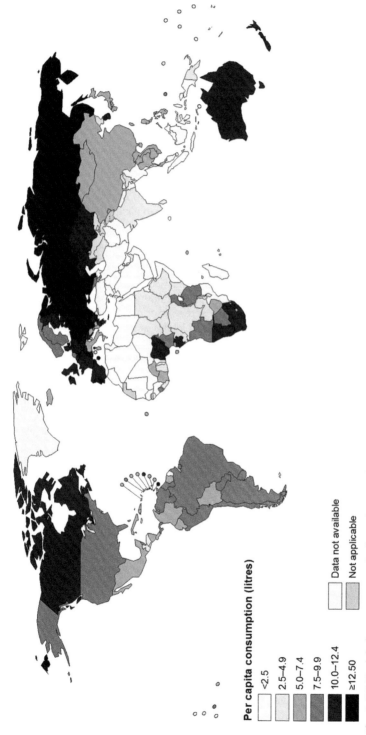

Per capita consumption (litres)

- <2.5
- 2.5–4.9
- 5.0–7.4
- 7.5–9.9
- 10.0–12.4
- ≥12.50
- Data not available
- Not applicable

Fig. 1. WHO global status report. The boundaries and names shown and the designations used on this map do not imply the expression of any opinion on the part of the World Health Organization concerning the legal status of any county, territory, city, or area or of its authorities, or concerning the delimitation of its frontiers or boundaries. Dotted and dashed lines on maps represent approximate border lines for which there may not yet be full agreement. (*From* World Health Organization. WHO global status report on alcohol and health. 2014. p. 29; with permission; *Data from* World Health Organization Map Production: Health Statistics and Information Systems (HSI). Geneva, Switzerland: World Health Organization; 2014.)

Table 1 Alcohol content by volume (ABV) of beverages in the United States				
Type of Beverage	ABV (%)	Standard Drink	Home (g)	Bar/Restaurant (g)
Beer	1–10.9	14 g (12 oz, ABV 5%)	12.8	17
Wine	7–13	14 g (5 oz, ABV 12%)	15.6	20
Liquor	35–60	14 g (1.5 oz, ABV 40%)	19.6	18.4

Standard drink definitions vary across countries and often contain less alcohol than the actual drinks poured. In the United States, a standard drink is considered to contain 14 g of alcohol. In Europe, a standard drink has 10 to 12 g. The ABV percentage and pour size may vary dramatically. As a result, drinkers often underestimate their alcohol intake.

Data from Kerr WC, Stockwell T. Understanding standard drinks and drinking guidelines. Drug Alcohol Rev 2012;31(2):200–5.

Mestizo peoples.[17] In white Europeans, the PNPLA3 polymorphism is more common in patients with ALD compared with controls and is significantly associated with the presence of steatosis, fibrosis, and cirrhosis.[18]

Drinking Patterns, Alcohol Intake, and Alcoholic Liver Injury

Although there is a strong correlation between per capita alcohol consumption and alcohol-related mortality, not all individuals who consume excessive amounts of alcohol develop ALD. The Dionysus cohort study surveyed 6534 Italians regarding alcohol intake.[7] Study subjects were screened for ALD and cirrhosis and followed for 3 years. Those individuals with a daily intake of greater than 30 g of alcohol had an increased risk of alcoholic liver injury and cirrhosis; those who consumed greater than 120 g of alcohol each day were most likely to develop cirrhosis, with an odds ratio of 62.3. However, even in the group with the highest alcohol intake, the overall prevalence of ALD was low (13.5%). In an autopsy study of 210 men, alcohol consumption of 40 to 80 g/d was associated with an increase in the frequency of hepatic steatosis from 11.7% to 42.7% and, for those who consumed greater than 80 g of alcohol per day, the incidence of advanced fibrosis and cirrhosis was significantly increased (relative risk = 8.8).[19]

Individuals who develop ALD are more likely to have started drinking at an early age and to have increased their alcohol consumption over the years.[20] In the United Kingdom, daily or near-daily heavy drinking, rather than binge or episodic drinking, was associated with increased rates of alcoholic liver injury.

NATURAL HISTORY OF ALCOHOLIC LIVER DISEASE

The diagnosis of ALD is based on a compatible clinical history, exclusion of other causes of liver disease, and histologic confirmation of characteristic findings. The spectrum of ALD includes simple steatosis, acute alcoholic hepatitis, and alcoholic cirrhosis (**Fig. 2**). There is frequent overlap of clinical and pathologic findings in affected patients.

Simple Steatosis

The development of fatty liver may occur in up to 90% of heavy drinkers and it can appear within 3 to 7 days of initial heavy alcohol consumption.[21] This condition typically is asymptomatic with normal or mildly increased serum aminotransferase levels and gamma-glutamyltransferase. Characteristic histologic findings of fatty liver include large-droplet steatosis in the centrilobular zone without significant inflammation or necrosis, although in severe cases the entire lobule may be

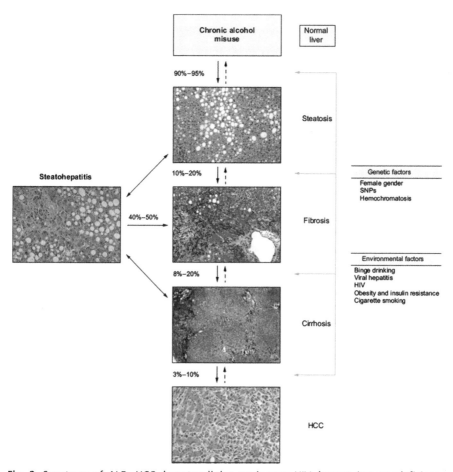

Fig. 2. Spectrum of ALD. HCC, hepatocellular carcinoma; HIV, human immunodeficiency virus; SNP, single nucleotide polymorphism. (*From* European Association for the Study of the Liver. EASL clinical practical guidelines: management of alcoholic liver disease. J Hepatol 2012;57:405; with permission.)

involved. The presence of simple steatosis on liver biopsy is no longer considered a benign condition. In a retrospective study of 88 patients with a histologic diagnosis of alcoholic fatty liver without alcoholic hepatitis or perivenular fibrosis, 18% of subjects progressed to fibrosis or cirrhosis over a median follow-up of 10.5 years.[9] In addition to the clinical risk factors of female gender and continued excessive alcohol use (40 units per week or the equivalent of 45 g/d), the presence of megamitochondria and mixed large-droplet and small-droplet steatosis on index biopsy were independently associated with development of fibrosis or cirrhosis.

Perivenular fibrosis may appear during the fatty liver stage of disease and correlates with higher levels of alcohol consumption.[22] This characteristic finding has subsequently been shown to be a precursor lesion of cirrhosis, and those individuals with perivenular fibrosis on index biopsy seem significantly more likely to develop advanced fibrosis in the setting of continued alcohol use.[23,24]

Alcoholic Foamy Degeneration

Alcoholic foamy degeneration is an uncommon entity characterized by jaundice, hepatomegaly, hyperlipidemia, and marked increase of serum aminotransferase, bilirubin, and alkaline phosphatase levels in the setting of chronic alcohol abuse.[25] Histologic evaluation reveals normal lobular architecture with perivenular fibrosis, hepatocyte swelling caused by accumulation of small-droplet fat, and megamitochondria. It is distinguished from alcoholic hepatitis by the absence of peripheral leukocytosis and inflammatory infiltrates on liver biopsy. Alcohol cessation is associated with complete recovery.[26]

Alcoholic Hepatitis

Alcoholic hepatitis is estimated to occur in 10% to 35% of heavy drinkers and has a poor prognosis.[1] Individuals with alcoholic hepatitis may present with mild, asymptomatic disease manifested by hepatomegaly and increased serum aminotransferase levels with the aspartate aminotransferase level twice or greater than the ALT level.[27] Severe disease is associated with jaundice, fever, malaise, tender hepatomegaly, and malnutrition. Affected individuals may develop ascites, hepatic encephalopathy, and hepatorenal syndrome. Pathologic features of severe alcoholic hepatitis include Mallory hyaline, ballooned hepatocytes, and a neutrophil-predominant inflammatory infiltrate.[21] The presence of perisinusoidal chicken-wire fibrosis as well as perivenular fibrosis is a distinctive feature of steatohepatitis. Short-term mortality may be as high as 50% in 30 days in patients with severe alcoholic hepatitis. A variety of prognostic tools have been developed to guide care for these individuals, including the Maddrey Discriminant Function, Model for End-stage Liver Disease (MELD) score, the Lille Model, and the Glasgow Alcoholic Hepatitis Score.[28–30] For more information on prognostic tools, please see Pierre M. Gholam: Prognosis and Prognostic Scoring Models for Alcoholic Liver Disease and Acute Alcoholic Hepatitis, in this issue.

An estimated 50% of individuals who enter hospital for treatment of acute alcoholic hepatitis have underlying cirrhosis at the time of presentation.[1] In addition, individuals with alcoholic hepatitis have a significantly increased risk of developing cirrhosis; studies have found development of cirrhosis during 4 to 8 years of follow-up in 27% of those who initially had mild alcoholic hepatitis and in 68% of those who had severe alcoholic hepatitis.[31] Despite alcohol cessation, most of the patients followed for 18 months by one investigator had persistent alcoholic hepatitis and 18% had developed cirrhosis.[32]

Alcoholic Cirrhosis

Cirrhosis is the 12th most common cause of death in the United States.[11] Alcohol remains the second most common cause of cirrhosis in the developed world, although determining the exact burden of disease is difficult. Although there is a consensus that alcohol is hepatotoxic and that excessive alcohol consumption increases the risk of developing cirrhosis, there is no clear dose-dependent relationship between drinking alcohol and development of alcoholic cirrhosis. A meta-analysis of 15 studies of alcohol intake and cirrhosis found a dose-response relationship between alcohol consumption and the risk of developing cirrhosis.[33] Even low-level alcohol intake (<25 g/d) was associated with a relative risk of cirrhosis ranging from 1.5 to 3.6. In another study of individuals without hepatitis B or C, the relative risk of liver cirrhosis was 44.7 among those with greater than 100 g of lifetime daily alcohol intake compared with those consuming significantly less alcohol.[34]

Additional causes of liver injury further increase the potential for development of cirrhosis in patients with ALD. For example, the combination of excessive alcohol intake and hepatitis C virus infection has a multiplicative effect on the risk of developing cirrhosis.[34] Obesity, a known cause of steatohepatitis, also seems to potentiate the effects of alcohol on fibrosis progression. In a large prospective cohort study of Scottish men, the presence of a high body mass index (BMI) and excess alcohol consumption had a supra-additive effect on the risk of liver disease morbidity and mortality, with a relative excess risk of 5.58 caused by this interaction of obesity and alcohol intake.[35] Individuals hospitalized for alcohol abuse or ALD who were overweight (BMI ≥25 in women, BMI ≥27 in men) for more than 10 years had a significantly higher risk of cirrhosis (60%) than nonoverweight patients (35%).[36]

A continuous cycle of injury and repair in patients with ALD results in deposition of collagen bands between portal areas and central veins that entrap nodules of hepatocytes. Resultant alcoholic cirrhosis is often characterized by small regenerative nodules, and is described as being micronodular.

Alcohol abstinence is critical even after diagnosis of cirrhosis, because abstinence significantly improves long-term prognosis. In a study of 100 patients with biopsy-proven alcoholic cirrhosis, abstinence at 1 month after diagnosis was the most significant predictor of long-term survival. The 7-year survival of patients who stopped drinking was 72% compared with 44% in those who continued to drink.[37] In hospitalized patients with cirrhosis, active alcohol intake was independently associated with a significant increase in the risk of death 5 years after discharge.[38] Overall, 5-year survival in patients with compensated cirrhosis who continue to drink is approximately 35%.

SUMMARY

Alcohol consumption and its harmful effects have increased over time, with the greatest socioeconomic and health burden in the developed world. Although there is no predictive formula for the quantity of alcohol people can safely drink, there is an expanding knowledge of risk factors, including genes that increase susceptibility to ALD such as PNPLA3. Through the excellent understanding of the broad spectrum of ALD and its related social and demographic context, clinicians can identify early and treat aggressively those affected individuals. It is hoped that, in the future, this awareness will allow physicians and patients to halt the process of liver injury in ALD and reverse some of its adverse consequences.

REFERENCES

1. O'Shea RS, Dasarathy S, McCullough AJ, Practice Guideline Committee of the American Association for the Study of Liver Diseases, Practice Parameters Committee of the American College of Gastroenterology. Alcoholic liver disease. Hepatology 2010;51(1):307–28.
2. World Health Organization. WHO global status report on alcohol and health. 2014. p. 1–100.
3. Mandayam S, Jamal MM, Morgan T. Epidemiology of alcoholic liver disease. Semin Liver Dis 2004;24(3):217–32.
4. Kim WR, Brown RS Jr, Terrault NA, et al. Burden of liver disease in the United States: summary of a workshop. Hepatology 2002;36(1):227–42.
5. Rehm J, Dawson D, Frick U, et al. Burden of disease associated with alcohol use disorders in the United States. Alcohol Clin Exp Res 2014;38(4):1068–77.
6. Oslin D. Late-life alcoholism: issues relevant to the geriatric psychiatrist. Am J Geriatr Psychiatry 2004;12(6):571–83.

7. Bellentani S, Saccoccio G, Costa G, et al, Dionysus Study Group. Drinking habits as cofactors of risk for alcohol induced liver damage. Gut 1997;41:845–50.
8. Becker U, Deis A, Sørensen TI, et al. Prediction of risk of liver disease by alcohol intake, sex, and age: a prospective population study. Hepatology 1996;23(5): 1025–9.
9. Teli MR, Day CP, Burt AD, et al. Determinants of progression to cirrhosis or fibrosis in pure alcoholic fatty liver. Lancet 1995;346:987–90.
10. Stinson FS, Grant BF, Dufour MC. The critical dimension of ethnicity in liver cirrhosis mortality statistics. Alcohol Clin Exp Res 2001;25(8):1181–7.
11. Yoon YH, Yi HY, Thomson PC. Liver cirrhosis mortality in the United States, 1970-2009, surveillance Report #93. National Institute on Alcohol Abuse and Alcoholism; 2012.
12. Levy RE, Catana AM, Durbin-Johnson B, et al. Ethnic differences in presentation and severity of alcoholic liver disease. Alcohol Clin Exp Res 2015;39(3):566–74.
13. Landen M, Roeber J, Naimi T, et al. Alcohol-attributable mortality among American Indians and Alaska natives in the United States, 1999–2009. Am J Public Health 2014;104:S343–9.
14. Romeo S, Kozlitina J, Xing C, et al. Genetic variation in PNPLA3 confers susceptibility to nonalcoholic fatty liver disease. Nat Genet 2008;40(12):1461–5.
15. Salameh H, Raff E, Erwin A, et al. PNPLA3 gene polymorphism is associated with predisposition to and severity of alcoholic liver disease. Am J Gastroenterol 2015; 110(6):846–56.
16. Pontoriero AC, Trinks J, Hulaniuk ML, et al. Influence of ethnicity on the distribution of genetic polymorphisms associated with risk of chronic liver disease in South American populations. BMC Genet 2015;16(1):93.
17. Larrieta-Carrasco E, Acuña-Alonzo V, Velázquez-Cruz R, et al. PNPLA3 I148M polymorphism is associated with elevated alanine transaminase levels in Mexican indigenous and Mestizo populations. Mol Biol Rep 2014;41(7):4705–11.
18. Trépo E, Gustot T, Degré D, et al. Common polymorphism in the PNPLA3/adiponutrin gene confers higher risk of cirrhosis and liver damage in alcoholic liver disease. J Hepatol 2011;55(4):906–12.
19. Savolainen VT, Liesto K, Männikkö A, et al. Alcohol consumption and alcoholic liver disease: evidence of a threshold level of effects of ethanol. Alcohol Clin Exp Res 1993;17(5):1112–7.
20. Hatton J, Burton A, Nash H, et al. Drinking patterns, dependency and life-time drinking history in alcohol-related liver disease. Addiction 2009;104(4):587–92.
21. Fleming KA, McGee JO. Alcohol induced liver disease. J Clin Pathol 1984;37: 721–33.
22. Savolainen V, Perola M, Lalu K, et al. Early perivenular fibrogenesis–precirrhotic lesions among moderate alcohol consumers and chronic alcoholics. J Hepatol 1995;23:S24–231.
23. Nakano M, Worner TM, Lieber CS. Perivenular fibrosis in alcoholic liver injury: ultrastructure and histologic progression. Gastroenterology 1982;83(4):777–85.
24. Worner TM, Lieber CS. Perivenular fibrosis as precursor lesion of cirrhosis. JAMA 1985;254(5):627–30.
25. Uchida T, Kao H, Quispe-Sjogren M, et al. Alcoholic foamy degeneration–a pattern of acute alcoholic injury of the liver. Gastroenterology 1983;84(4):683–92.
26. Ruiz P, Michelena J, Altamirano J, et al. Hepatic hemodynamics and transient elastography in alcoholic foamy degeneration: report of 2 cases. Ann Hepatol 2012;11(3):399–403.
27. Sass DA, Shaikh OS. Alcoholic hepatitis. Clin Liver Dis 2006;10:219–37.

28. Dunn W, Jamil LH, Brown LS, et al. MELD accurately predicts mortality in patients with alcoholic hepatitis. Hepatology 2005;41(2):353–8.
29. Forrest EH, Evans CD, Stewart S, et al. Analysis of factors predictive of mortality in alcoholic hepatitis and derivation and validation of the Glasgow alcoholic hepatitis score. Gut 2005;54:1174–9.
30. Maddrey WC, Boitnott JK, Bedine MS, et al. Corticosteroid therapy of alcoholic hepatitis. Gastroenterology 1978;75(2):193–9.
31. Bird GLA, Williams R. Factors determining cirrhosis in alcoholic liver disease. Mol Aspects Med 1988;10:97–105.
32. Galambos J. Natural history of alcoholic hepatitis. 3. Histological changes. Gastroenterology 1972;63(6):1026–35.
33. Corrao G, Bagnardi V, Zambon A, et al. Meta-analysis of alcohol intake in relation to risk of liver cirrhosis. Alcohol 1998;33(4):381–92.
34. Corrao G, Aricò S. Independent and combined action of hepatitis C virus infection and alcohol consumption on the risk of symptomatic liver cirrhosis. Hepatology 1998;27:914–9.
35. Hart CL, Morrison DS, Batty GD, et al. Effect of body mass index and alcohol consumption on liver disease: analysis of data from two prospective cohort studies. Br Med J 2010;11:1–7.
36. Naveau S, Giraud V, Borotto E, et al. Excess weight risk factor for alcoholic liver disease. Hepatology 1997;25(108–111):108–11.
37. Verrill C, Markham H, Templeton A, et al. Alcohol-related cirrhosis–early abstinence is a key factor in prognosis, even in the most severe cases. Addiction 2009;104(5):768–74.
38. Pessione F, Ramond MJ, Peters L, et al. Five-year survival predictive factors in patients with excessive alcohol intake and cirrhosis. Effect of alcoholic hepatitis, smoking and abstinence. Liver Int 2003;23(1):45–53.

Unhealthy Alcohol Use

Stephen Holt, MD, MS[a],*, Jeanette Tetrault, MD[b]

KEYWORDS

- Alcoholism • Alcohol use disorder • Addiction • Screening • Diagnosis
- Brief intervention • Pharmacotherapy

KEY POINTS

- Unhealthy alcohol use, which encompasses the spectrum of alcohol consumption from at-risk drinking to alcohol use disorder, is common and routine screening is an essential strategy to identify patients and initiate appropriate treatment.
- At-risk drinking can be managed with brief interventions, which is a counseling strategy designed to enhance patients' motivations and promote behavioral change.
- Alcohol withdrawal can be managed in the inpatient or outpatient setting, preferably with benzodiazepines using a symptom-triggered approach.
- Decades of research now support the use of several US Food and Drug Administration–approved medications for the treatment of alcohol use disorder, aiding in promoting abstinence and reducing heavy drinking days.

INTRODUCTION

Unhealthy alcohol use ranges from use that puts patients at risk of health consequences to use causing multiple medical and/or behavioral problems meeting Diagnostic and Statistical Manual of Mental Disorders, Fifth Edition (DSM-V) diagnostic criteria for alcohol use disorder (AUD). In the United States, more than 79,000 deaths a year are attributed to unhealthy alcohol use, with roughly 1 in 10 deaths among working-aged adults resulting from excessive drinking.[1] The annual economic cost of alcohol use in the United States is estimated to be more than $220 billion. Thus, alcohol and its associated health problems have a major impact on the practices of generalist and specialty providers.[2,3]

Patients with unhealthy alcohol use present several unique challenges for providers.[4] As with other chronic diseases, unhealthy alcohol use ranges from asymptomatic to severe and providers should be able to recognize and treat patients at all points in the spectrum of disease. This article outlines screening and assessment with an emphasis on the use of appropriate terminology, and discusses available treatment options.

Disclosure: The authors have nothing to disclose.
[a] Section of General Internal Medicine, Department of Medicine, Yale School of Medicine, 1450 Chapel Street, New Haven, CT 06511, USA; [b] Section of General Internal Medicine, Department of Medicine, Yale School of Medicine, 367 Cedar Street, New Haven, CT 06510, USA
* Corresponding author.
E-mail address: Stephen.holt@yale.edu

Clin Liver Dis 20 (2016) 429–444
http://dx.doi.org/10.1016/j.cld.2016.02.003

liver.theclinics.com

DEFINITIONS AND CLASSIFICATION

When considering patients who may have alcohol-related problems, it is helpful to distinguish between 3 types of alcohol use: (1) moderate drinking; (2) at-risk drinking (often called hazardous drinking), which places patients at risk for alcohol-related problems; and (3) drinking with evidence of AUD (often called harmful drinking), which directly causes specific alcohol-related problems. The term unhealthy alcohol use refers to the spectrum of use encompassing at-risk drinking and AUD.[3]

Moderate Drinking

Moderate drinking is defined in terms of the average number of drinks consumed a day that places an adult at low risk for alcohol-related health problems (ie, not meeting criteria for at-risk drinking, defined later).[5] Although some evidence suggests that low levels of alcohol intake may have health benefits,[6,7] the degree to which moderate drinking may confer health benefits and may be associated with reduced mortality (specifically, reduction of cardiovascular mortality) remains controversial.[8]

At-Risk Drinking

At-risk drinking refers to consumption of an amount of alcohol that puts an individual at risk for health consequences. Individuals with at-risk alcohol use may go on to develop an AUD.[9] The National Institute on Alcohol Abuse and Alcoholism (NIAAA) in the United States has estimated consumption amounts of alcohol that increase health risks.[9] In men less than age 65 years, consumption of more than 14 standard drinks per week on average or more than 4 drinks per day, and, in women and adults 65 years and older, consumption of more than 7 standard drinks per week on average or more than 3 drinks on any day puts an individual at risk for health consequences. Specifying these thresholds is an inexact science based on epidemiologic evidence. Amounts are based on a standard drink, which is defined as 12 g of ethanol, as found in 148 mL (5 ounces) of wine, 355 mL (12 ounces) of beer, or 44 mL (1.5 ounces) of 40% (80-proof) spirits. Note that smaller amounts of regular alcohol use may constitute at-risk use in specific populations (eg, pregnant women, or people who experience alcohol-associated injuries or infection with a sexually transmitted diseases).

Synonyms for at-risk alcohol use include hazardous use and risky use. Heavy alcohol use, a related term without a well-specified, widely accepted definition, can refer to a pattern over time or to a single episode of heavy drinking. The term alcoholism, which is perhaps the most widely used term to describe patients with alcohol problems, has lost much of its usefulness because of the imprecision in its definition and the stigma associated with the term.

Alcohol Use Disorder

The DSM-V combines the previous constructs of alcohol abuse and alcohol dependence from the DSM-IV into a single disorder, AUD, measured on a continuum from mild to severe.[10] AUD is considered a maladaptive pattern of alcohol use leading to clinically significant impairment or distress, as manifested by 2 (or more) of 11 criteria, occurring within a 12-month period.

Binge Drinking

Binge drinking has been defined by the NIAAA as "drinking so much within about two hours that blood alcohol concentration (BAC) levels reach 0.08 g/dL."[9] In women, this typically occurs after about 4 standard drinks, and, in men, after about 5 standard drinks.

EPIDEMIOLOGY

In a 2002 survey, 60% of adults (72% of men) in the United States reported that they drink alcohol. Alcohol-related problems are common in the general population; however, the prevalence of these problems has varied with different studies. The Centers for Disease Control and Prevention reported that, in 2012, approximately 17% of US adults (38 million individuals) reported binge drinking. Studies have shown that unhealthy alcohol use is highly prevalent, especially in patients presenting to general medical practices. For example, in 2 intervention studies, at-risk drinking was identified in 41% of men and 28% of women from 47 general practices in the United Kingdom[11] and in 1 in 6 patients in 17 general practices in the United States.[12] In various studies of outpatients, the lifetime prevalence of AUD ranged from 13% to 22%.[13–16]

GENETICS AND ENVIRONMENT

Evidence from family, twin, and adoption studies supports a strong genetic component for the risk of AUD.[17,18] In general, most studies of twins have shown a higher concordance of AUD in monozygotic twins than in dizygotic twins. Adoption studies generally document that adopted children with a biological parent with an AUD have a 2-fold to 3-fold greater risk of AUD than adopted children whose biological parents do not have an AUD.[19] Although genetic predisposition is clearly a major risk factor for alcohol-related problems, environmental influences may also impart risk. Such environmental influences include negative life events, occupational stress, expectancies about alcohol, personality factors (eg, problem-prone behavior during adolescence), and interpersonal influences (eg, the behaviors of family members or peers).[18,20] A body of research also suggests that certain genetic factors may dictate response to medications used to treat AUD, as outlined later.

COMMON PROBLEMS ASSOCIATED WITH ALCOHOL USE DISORDER

Familiarity with the wide variety of medical, behavioral, and psychiatric complications of heavy drinking or AUD facilitates detection and management of alcohol-related problems in patients.

Medical Problems

The numerous medical complications associated with excessive alcohol consumption have been well documented.[3,21] Patients may present to physicians with acute and chronic clinical signs and symptoms that are the direct or indirect results of alcohol use. The most common medical effects of alcohol are seen in the central and peripheral nervous systems.[22] These effects are intoxication, withdrawal, seizures, delirium and dementia, stroke, and peripheral neuropathy. Similarly, alcohol has a wide variety of effects on the gastrointestinal system, including esophageal diseases (eg, Mallory-Weiss tears), gastritis, and peptic ulcer disease.[23] Liver diseases, including acute alcoholic hepatitis and cirrhosis, are also highly prevalent.[24] In addition, patients with alcohol-related liver disease are at increased risk for hepatotoxicity from medications and herbal supplements.[25] Alcohol use may also worsen the clinical outcomes in patients with other causes of liver disease, such as viral hepatitis, and nonalcoholic fatty liver disease.[26] Acute and chronic pancreatic disease is also a common manifestation of alcohol use.[27]

Patients with chronic alcohol use may experience a wide range of cardiovascular effects, such as hypertension, left ventricular hypertrophy, cardiomyopathy, arrhythmias, and sudden death.[28,29] In contrast, moderate alcohol consumption has been associated with a decreased risk of coronary heart disease and improved prognosis after myocardial infarction.[30,31]

Along with causing major neurologic, digestive system, and cardiovascular effects, alcohol use is associated with a variety of other organ-based effects. Heavy alcohol use is associated with cancer of the upper digestive and respiratory tracts, the liver, and other organs.[32] Alcohol use has also been associated with metabolic, endocrine, and rheumatologic abnormalities, such as osteoporosis, menstrual dysfunction, male hypogonadism, thyroid and adrenal dysfunction, and gout.[33,34] Binge drinking, heavy weekly alcohol consumption, and drinking while underage or pregnant, has also been found to result in 1 in 10 deaths among working-age adults.[1]

Psychiatric Problems

Epidemiologic surveys have shown high rates of psychiatric illness in persons diagnosed with AUD, and comorbid psychiatric disease is associated with increased health care use in patients with alcohol-related problems.[35,36] Patients with depression have a higher prevalence of concurrent AUD than the general population.[37] In addition, suicide risk has been shown to increase with increasing levels of alcohol use.[38]

Other Behavior-Related Problems

Unhealthy alcohol use can harm persons other than the user; it has been linked to increased rates of accidents and injuries, violence against others, and spousal abuse.[39–41] Unhealthy alcohol use is also linked to other high-risk behaviors (eg, drug and tobacco use and high-risk sexual activity) that carry increased risk of disease. Alcohol use is commonly encountered in association with other substance use disorders, including abuse of prescription drugs.[42]

SCREENING AND ASSESSMENT

Despite the prevalence of alcohol-related problems and their impact on health, most studies show that unhealthy alcohol use is not routinely detected in medical settings.[43] AUD is most likely to be identified in patients experiencing severe medical complications, such as alcoholic hepatitis or cirrhosis.[16] Earlier detection of at-risk drinking before the onset of organ damage or of AUD may be critical in preventing late sequelae.

Screening for unhealthy alcohol use should be incorporated into the routine care of all patients.[4] The first step is to inquire about current and past alcohol use in all patients. Current recommendations are to screen with a single question: "How many times in the past year have you had 5 or more drinks in a day (for men less than 65 years old; 4 or more drinks in a day for women or anyone more than 65 years old)?" It is recommended that individuals who screen negative be queried about past problems with alcohol and receive advice regarding drinking limits (discussed earlier) or abstinence, as indicated (pregnancy, medical problems exacerbated by alcohol, medications that interact with alcohol). In individuals with a positive screen for unhealthy alcohol use in response to the single question, recommendations are to follow up with questions regarding the weekly average. Because treatment recommendations differ for those who meet criteria for at-risk drinking and those with AUD, the second step involves determining the presence or absence of AUD as outlined by the DSM-V criteria.

The assessment for evidence of specific alcohol-related medical and psychiatric problems should include a thorough history and physical examination. Although not useful as screening tests for AUD, laboratory tests, such as liver enzyme assay, may be useful in identifying undiagnosed alcohol-related medical problems.[32] In addition, knowledge of previous treatment of alcohol-related problems is essential when referring patients for treatment.

TREATMENT APPROACHES FOR PATIENTS WITH UNHEALTHY ALCOHOL USE

As outlined earlier, the spectrum of unhealthy alcohol use ranges from at-risk drinking to severe AUD. Across this spectrum, the severity of disease dictates the most appropriate level of behavioral and pharmacologic treatment approaches. Patients at the more severe end of this spectrum are likely to require care from an addiction specialist, although primary care physicians or other specialists can still play a critical role in the management of their patients with unhealthy alcohol use, regardless of severity. This role may include screening and diagnosis; evaluating patients for complications of alcohol use; aiding in enhancing patients' motivation to change their patterns of drinking; providing support for ongoing treatments; and, importantly, monitoring patients for relapse. Moreover, it behooves primary care providers and other non–addiction medicine specialist providers alike to gain familiarity with the growing list of available medications for treating AUD, all of which have established safety profiles, are effective, and are grossly underused.[44–46]

The first step in creating a treatment plan for patients showing unhealthy alcohol use is to assess the patient's readiness to embrace change. Patients with unhealthy drinking patterns may show denial or ambivalence about their drinking, which can lead to resistance to any proposed treatment plans. One well-established model for conceptualizing patients' readiness to change describes 6 stages along a continuum, from a precontemplation stage, in which the patient is unaware of or unaccepting of the alcohol problem, to a more contemplative stage when the patient is more likely to benefit from treatment option discussions (**Table 1**).[47] Having assessed the patient's readiness to change, the health care provider should next attempt to steer the patient further along the readiness continuum, by enhancing the patient's motivations to change. This process can be done by any health care provider, using a technique known as brief intervention (BI) therapy.[48–50]

Table 1
Stages of readiness to change addictive behaviors and stage-specific approaches

Stage	Patient Features	Possible Approaches
Precontemplation	Unaware of alcohol problems	Express concern about health problems and their link to alcohol use
Contemplation	Recognizes alcohol problems	Reinforce links between alcohol use and problems; promote behavior change
Determination	Decides to change behavior	Support decision; provide advice about short-term and long-term actions to change behavior
Action	Changes behavior	Monitor compliance with advice and outcomes
Maintenance	Continues new behavior	Continue follow-up of alcohol problems; support behavior change and treatment efforts; monitor for relapse
Relapse	Recurrence of alcohol problems	Support return to behavior change or reentry into or continuation of treatment; monitor for alcohol problems

Adapted from DiClemente CC, Bellino LE, Neavins TM. Motivation for change and alcoholism treatment. Alcohol Res Health 1999;23(2):86.

MANAGEMENT OF AT-RISK DRINKERS WITH BRIEF INTERVENTION THERAPY

BIs are counseling sessions of 5 to 20 minutes, conducted on 1 or more occasions. They are effective when used by generalist and specialist physicians alike, and their use in primary care settings has been promoted by experts and government agencies.[50–53] A BI begins with first asking the patient's permission to further discuss the patient's drinking. Having obtained permission, the provider next attempts to elicit from the patient the perceived benefits and risks of continuing to drink at current levels, helping the patient as needed to identify potential links between the patient's alcohol use and any alcohol-related problems. The provider should clearly state how the patient's drinking patterns compare with currently recommended limits. The FRAMES (feedback, responsibility, advice, menu, empathy, self-efficacy) acronym (**Box 1**) describes a counseling strategy commonly used while conducting a BI.[49] If the patient expresses any interest in reducing alcohol intake, the provider can then present a menu of treatment options and then aid the patient in defining explicit, achievable drinking goals that can be followed up at the next visit. In contrast, patients who continue to express reluctance to make any changes can be merely thanked for their willingness to openly discuss their personal habits.

The impact of BI, and the ideal frequency and duration of interventions, has been extensively studied. A comprehensive systematic review and meta-analysis funded by the Agency for Healthcare Research and Quality identified 23 controlled trials studying the impact of various counseling interventions on unhealthy alcohol use.[50] The analysis found that brief (10–15 minutes), multicontact interventions were the most effective

---

Box 1
Components of a brief intervention

FRAMES Counseling strategy for BI

Feedback
  Review the problems experienced by the patient because of alcohol use

Responsibility
  Emphasize that changing patterns of alcohol use is the patient's choice and responsibility

Advice
  Advise the patient to cut down or abstain from alcohol

Menu
  Provide menu of options and strategies for changing behavior

Empathy
  Use a warm, empathic, understanding approach with the patient

Self-efficacy
  Encourage optimism about likelihood and benefits of changing behavior

Specific brief intervention therapeutic techniques

Workbook with feedback on health behavior

Review of the prevalence of problem drinking and adverse effects of alcohol

Worksheet on drinking cues

Drinking agreement prescription

Drinking diary

Adapted from Miller WR, Rollnick S. Motivational interviewing: preparing people to change addictive behavior. New York: The Guilford Press; 1991; with permission.

strategy to decrease alcohol consumption in patients showing at-risk or harmful drinking, with a 12% decrease in reported heavy drinking days (risk difference, 0.12; confidence interval [CI], 0.07–0.12). This study, along with others, shows that simple BIs can effectively reduce patients' at-risk drinking behaviors, and are within the scope of non–addiction specialists.[48,54,55] In contrast, there are limited data to support the efficacy of BI in reducing drinking in patients with more severe AUD.[55]

MANAGEMENT OF ALCOHOL USE DISORDERS

Although patients with at-risk drinking may only require BI and close follow-up, those with AUD may experience significant complications that necessitate more intensive treatment. Non–addiction specialist clinicians may be called on to initiate this more intensive treatment, which may include the management of alcohol withdrawal syndrome (AWS); initial pharmacotherapy to minimize cravings and reduce the risk of relapse; and, when necessary, referral to an alcohol treatment program or addiction specialist.

Alcohol Withdrawal Syndrome

When people accustomed to heavy drinking abruptly discontinue or significantly cut back on their use, a constellation of signs and symptoms may ensue over the subsequent hours and days. These symptoms may include mild withdrawal symptoms in the first 24 hours, including tremors, anxiety, nausea, insomnia, and headache. These symptoms may then progress to severe alcohol withdrawal after 3 to 5 days, with concomitant autonomic instability, increases in adrenergic tone, more significant gastrointestinal symptoms, and profound central nervous system effects (eg, agitation, hallucinations, seizures, and delirium tremens). The symptoms of alcohol withdrawal, and the impact of ongoing treatments, may be objectively assessed over time using the well-validated revised Clinical Institute Withdrawal Assessment for Alcohol, Revised (CIWA-Ar) protocol.[56] Several patient factors have been identified that increase the likelihood that a particular patient is at high risk of developing severe AWS. These factors include increased baseline blood pressure, significant medical or psychiatric comorbidities, and previous complicated withdrawal.[57] Pecoraro and colleagues[58] found that the Alcohol Use Disorders Identification Test-(Piccinelli) Consumption (AUDIT-PC), an abbreviated 5-item version of the widely used 10-item AUDIT screening tool, had excellent discriminating ability for predicting which patients admitted to the hospital were likely to develop AWS (**Table 2**). Using a cutoff score of greater than or equal to 4, the investigators found a sensitivity of 91.0% and specificity 89.7% (area under the curve, 0.95; 95% CI, 0.94–0.97) for predicting AWS; performance characteristics that were subsequently validated in a sensitivity analysis.

The management of AWS is geared toward minimizing complications (eg, seizures, delirium, intubation), while mitigating the potential side effects of CNS-acting medications. Although countless medications have been studied for the pharmacologic management of AWS, the mainstay of treatment remains the benzodiazepines, which have been consistently shown to be the safest and most effective medications for this purpose.[59,60] Many reviews have suggested that the longer-acting benzodiazepines provide a smoother withdrawal and may be more effective in preventing seizure, whereas shorter-acting benzodiazepines with fewer active metabolites are considered to be safer in the elderly and in patients with severe liver disease.[60,61] When used in the treatment and prevention of AWS, benzodiazepines are best used via a symptom-triggered approach, in which benzodiazepines are administered according to a protocolized scoring system (eg, the CIWA-Ar) that dictates dosing schedules as needed for

Table 2
The AUDIT-PC

Questions	Scoring System					Score
	0	1	2	3	4	
How often do you have a drink containing alcohol?	Never	Monthly or less	2–4 times per month	2–3 times per week	4+ times per week	
How many units of alcohol do you drink on a typical day when you are drinking?	1–2	3–4	5–6	7–9	10+	
How often during the last year have you found that you were not able to stop drinking once you had started?	Never	Less than monthly	Monthly	Weekly	Daily or almost daily	
How often during the last year have you failed to do what was normally expected from you because of your drinking?	Never	Less than monthly	Monthly	Weekly	Daily or almost daily	
Has a relative or friend, doctor, or other health worker been concerned about your drinking or suggested that you cut down?	No	—	Yes, but not in the last year	—	Yes, during the last year	

An AUDIT-PC score of 4 or greater predicts impending AWS in newly hospitalized patients.
Adapted from Pecoraro A, Ewen E, Horton T, et al, Using the AUDIT-PC to predict alcohol withdrawal in hospitalized patients. J Gen Intern Med 2014;29(1):35; with permission.

objective signs and symptoms of ongoing withdrawal. Ongoing research continues to investigate the potential utility of other adjunctive, nonbenzodiazepine medications such as dexmedetomidine, phenobarbital, carbamazepine, gabapentin, and ketamine for the treatment of AWS, although larger studies are needed.[60,62–65] In addition, it is critical to begin the process of planning for posthospital treatment early in the patient's hospital stay to help maintain abstinence after discharge.

Many patients with AUD can be treated safely and effectively in the outpatient environment after treatment of AWS, if necessary, is completed.[66] The National Institute for Health and Clinical Excellence has defined criteria that may aid clinicians in decisions regarding patient placement.[61] Clinical variables that are important in determining the level of service needed include the presence of medical or psychiatric comorbidity, the risk of withdrawal, the level of social support available, and previous treatment experience.

PSYCHOTHERAPEUTIC APPROACHES TO THE TREATMENT OF ALCOHOL DEPENDENCE

Behavioral interventions for AUD may include BI (described earlier), intensive outpatient programs with individual or group therapy sessions, 12-step programs such as Alcoholics Anonymous (AA), and newer technology-based approaches (eg, text messaging systems) to promote abstinence and recovery.[67] These approaches vary based on the particular resources in a given community, the skillset of the treatment team, and the preferences of specific patients. In light of the complex biopsychosocial factors that contribute to addictive disorders, behavioral interventions typically continue for months to years, although they may become less intensive as patients progress through stages of recovery. Well-studied psychotherapeutic approaches include cognitive-behavioral coping skills therapy, motivational-enhancement therapy, and 12-step facilitation, each of which has been shown to significantly increase the likelihood of maintaining prolonged abstinence.[68,69]

Self-Help Groups

AA and similar groups are based on a 12-step recovery model. In this model, 12 steps describe specific attitudes, beliefs, and actions that are regarded as critical to the recovery process. Meetings take place at multiple times of day, every day of the week, in multiple locations throughout the country and include both open meetings, which are open to everyone, and closed meetings, which are restricted to AA members (the only requirement is a desire to stop drinking). Studies have consistently shown that attendance at AA meetings correlates with positive drinking outcomes, including reductions in problem drinking and improved abstinence rates.[70–72] Moreover, the extent to which AA members participate in AA activities (ie, obtaining a program sponsor and frequency of meeting attendance) correlates highly with sustained abstinence rates.[71]

PHARMACOLOGIC TREATMENTS TO PREVENT RELAPSE

Despite the availability of well-studied, well-tolerated, and consistently effective pharmacotherapies for the treatment of AUD, less than one-quarter of patients with AUD ever receive treatment.[44,45] The United States Food and Drug Administration (FDA) has approved 4 medications for this purpose (**Table 3**): disulfiram, oral naltrexone, long-acting injectable naltrexone, and acamprosate. However, several other medications have promising data to support their use as well. A useful guide (TIP-49 [Treatment Improvement Protocol 49]) that reviews the FDA-approved medications for AUD was published by The Center for Substance Abuse Treatment in 2009, and is freely available at www.samhsa.gov.

Table 3
Pharmacotherapeutic agents for relapse prevention (FDA approved)

Drug	Starting Dose (mg)	Maintenance Dose (mg)	Interval	Comments
Disulfiram	125–500	125–500	Once a day in the morning	Requires careful patient education about disulfiram-alcohol interaction; used for abstinence
Naltrexone	50 (oral) 380 (IM)	50 380	Once a day Once a month	Contraindicated in patients taking opioids; side effects include nausea, headache, depression; may be used in those wishing to cut back on drinking
Acamprosate	666	666	Three times a day	Side effects include diarrhea and insomnia; best used when abstinence is the goal

Abbreviation: IM, intramuscular.

Disulfiram, typically prescribed as a once-daily dose of 500 mg, has been in clinical use since 1948.[73] As an acetaldehyde dehydrogenase inhibitor, disulfiram blocks the metabolism of acetaldehyde, the first downstream metabolite of alcohol, leading to a toxic accumulation of acetaldehyde. This action precipitates an unpleasant disulfiram reaction characterized by nausea, headache, dizziness, flushing, and palpitations. As such, disulfiram is only appropriate for patients intending to completely abstain from alcohol. A meta-analysis showed substantial benefits compared with controls on a set of alcohol primary end points (effect size $g = .70$; 95% CI, 0.46–0.93).[74] Nonetheless, this medication is best reserved for highly motivated patients, and ideally under conditions in which adherence to disulfiram can be closely monitored, either by a member of the clinical team or by a close friend or relative.

Naltrexone is an opioid antagonist that was originally developed for the treatment of opioid dependence, until it was subsequently found to be useful in treating AUD.[75] Available as a 50-mg oral tablet for daily dosing and a long-acting 380-mg injectable form taken intramuscularly once monthly, naltrexone has been shown to decrease alcohol's pleasurable effects and cravings associated with chronic use.[76] A large 2014 meta-analysis found that treatment with oral naltrexone, compared with placebo, was associated with a number needed to treat (NNT) of 12 to prevent a return to heavy drinking (95% CI, 9–26), whereas intramuscular naltrexone was associated with a significant reduction in the number of heavy drinking days per month (weighted mean difference, −4.6%; 95% CI, −8.5% to −0.56%).[77] Common side effects include nausea, headache, and depression. Although hepatotoxicity is rare, even when used in patients with other chronic conditions, it is reasonable to check liver function tests before and after starting naltrexone, although it has been safely used in patients with Child-Pugh class A or B cirrhosis.[78,79] The intramuscular form can lead to injection site reactions (pain, swelling, skin infection), but has the benefit of improved adherence. Both naltrexone formulations are contraindicated in patients taking prescription opioids.

Acamprosate, thought to work by restoring balance in the gamma-aminobutyric acid–ergic (GABAergic) and glutamatergic neurotransmitter systems, has been studied extensively.[77,80,81] A recent meta-analysis found that acamprosate yielded improvements in abstinence outcomes with an NNT of 12 in preventing return to any drinking, compared with placebo (95% CI, 8–26).[77] In comparisons between acamprosate and naltrexone, acamprosate seems to be superior at promoting absti-nence, whereas naltrexone is more effective at reducing heavy drinking.[81] Adherence is a significant issue with this medication because it is prescribed as two 333-mg tablets 3 times daily. Safe in patients with Child-Pugh class A and B cirrhosis, the most common side effect is diarrhea, occurring in as many as 16% of patients.[82] It is contraindicated in patients with renal dysfunction.

Among newer drugs not yet FDA approved for treating AUD, topiramate has shown considerable promise. In a recent meta-analysis, topiramate was effective at promot-ing abstinence (g = 0.468; $P<.01$), curbing heavy drinking (g = 0.406; $P<.01$), and reducing increases in the levels of hepatic enzyme gamma-glutamyl transferase (GGT) (g = 0.324; $P = .02$).[83] Topiramate is thought to act via its GABAergic and anti-glutamatergic properties. Unlike the aforementioned FDA-approved medications, achieving therapeutic doses of topiramate necessitates a gradual dose escalation over a period of 4 to 8 weeks to a goal regimen of 1 to 200 mg twice daily.[83,84] Possible unpleasant side effects include cognitive disturbances, gastrointestinal upset, taste perversion, and other paresthesias. Topiramate doses should be adjusted in patients with creatinine clearance less than 70 mL/min.

Additional medications under study with promising preliminary results include nalmefene (already approved for use in the European Union), varenicline, pregabalin, and gabapentin.[77,85–90]

SUMMARY

A wide body of research has furthered understanding of the myriad ways that un-healthy alcohol use can contribute to morbidity and mortality. With as many as 1 in 6 patients in the United States showing at-risk drinking, the first step in reducing the public health burden of unhealthy alcohol use is the routine screening of all pa-tients. Although patients with at-risk drinking may be managed by their health care providers using BIs, patients with AUD are likely to need more aggressive thera-pies. These therapies, tailored to each patient's individual needs, may include referral to a 12-step program, longitudinal behavioral therapy from a clinical psychologist or counselor, the outpatient or inpatient management of alcohol with-drawal with benzodiazepines, and/or longer-term treatment with one of several available pharmacotherapies. There are currently 4 FDA-approved medications with favorable safety profiles and efficacy data, as well as several off-label medications that show similar promise in the treatment of AUD. With significant advances in screening methods, behavioral strategies, and pharmacotherapies, it behooves both generalist and specialist clinicians to develop a familiarity with treatment options so that they might implement these treatments in their own practices.

REFERENCES

1. Stahre M, Roeber J, Kanny D, et al. Contribution of excessive alcohol consump-tion to deaths and years of potential life lost in the United States. Prev Chronic Dis 2014;11:E109.
2. Room R, Babor T, Rehm J. Alcohol and public health. Lancet 2005;365(9458): 519–30.
3. Saitz R. Clinical practice. Unhealthy alcohol use. N Engl J Med 2005;352(6): 596–607.
4. O'Connor PG, Schottenfeld RS. Patients with alcohol problems. N Engl J Med 1998;338(9):592–602.

5. Westermeyer J. A sea change in the treatment of alcoholism. Am J Psychiatry 2008;165(9):1093–5.

6. Knoops KT, de Groot LC, Kromhout D, et al. Mediterranean diet, lifestyle factors, and 10-year mortality in elderly European men and women: the HALE project. JAMA 2004;292(12):1433–9.

7. Mukamal KJ, Conigrave KM, Mittleman MA, et al. Roles of drinking pattern and type of alcohol consumed in coronary heart disease in men. N Engl J Med 2003;348(2):109–18.

8. Plunk AD, Syed-Mohammed H, Cavazos-Rehg P, et al. Alcohol consumption, heavy drinking, and mortality: rethinking the j-shaped curve. Alcohol Clin Exp Res 2014;38(2):471–8.

9. National Institute on Alcohol Abuse and Alcoholism (NIAAA). Helping patients who drink too much: a clinician's guide. Bethesda (MD): NIAAA; 2005.

10. American Psychiatric Association. Diagnostic and statistical manual. 5th edition. Arlington (VA): American Psychiatric Association; 2013.

11. Wallace P, Cutler S, Haines A. Randomised controlled trial of general practitioner intervention in patients with excessive alcohol consumption. BMJ 1988; 297(6649):663–8.

12. Fleming MF, Barry KL, Manwell LB, et al. Brief physician advice for problem alcohol drinkers. A randomized controlled trial in community-based primary care practices. JAMA 1997;277(13):1039–45.

13. Friedmann PD, Saitz R, Gogineni A, et al. Validation of the screening strategy in the NIAAA "Physicians' Guide to Helping Patients with Alcohol Problems. J Stud Alcohol 2001;62(2):234–8.

14. Holt SR, Ramos J, Harma MA, et al. Prevalence of unhealthy substance use on teaching and hospitalist medical services: implications for education. Am J Addict 2012;21(2):111–9.

15. McQuade WH, Levy SM, Yanek LR, et al. Detecting symptoms of alcohol abuse in primary care settings. Arch Fam Med 2000;9(9):814–21.

16. Moore RD, Bone LR, Geller G, et al. Prevalence, detection, and treatment of alcoholism in hospitalized patients. JAMA 1989;261(3):403–7.

17. Nestler EJ. Genes and addiction. Nat Genet 2000;26(3):277–81.

18. Schuckit MA. Genetics of the risk for alcoholism. Am J Addict 2000;9(2):103–12.

19. Nurnberger JI Jr, Wiegand R, Bucholz K, et al. A family study of alcohol dependence: coaggregation of multiple disorders in relatives of alcohol-dependent probands. Arch Gen Psychiatry 2004;61(12):1246–56.

20. Light JM, Irvine KM, Kjerulf L. Estimating genetic and environmental effects of alcohol use and dependence from a national survey: a "quasi-adoption" study. J Stud Alcohol 1996;57(5):507–20.

21. Magruder-Habib K, Durand AM, Frey KA. Alcohol abuse and alcoholism in primary health care settings. J Fam Pract 1991;32(4):406–13.

22. Charness ME, Simon RP, Greenberg DA. Ethanol and the nervous system. N Engl J Med 1989;321(7):442–54.

23. Fields JZ, Turk A, Durkin M, et al. Increased gastrointestinal symptoms in chronic alcoholics. Am J Gastroenterol 1994;89(3):382–6.

24. Lieber CS. Medical disorders of alcoholism. N Engl J Med 1995;333(16):1058–65.

25. Tanaka E, Yamazaki K, Misawa S. Update: the clinical importance of acetaminophen hepatotoxicity in non-alcoholic and alcoholic subjects. J Clin Pharm Ther 2000;25(5):325–32.

26. Aloman C, Gehring S, Wintermeyer P, et al. Chronic ethanol consumption impairs cellular immune responses against HCV NS5 protein due to dendritic cell dysfunction. Gastroenterology 2007;132(2):698–708.

27. Jaakkola M, Sillanaukee P, Löf K, et al. Amount of alcohol is an important determinant of the severity of acute alcoholic pancreatitis. Surgery 1994;115(1):31–8.

28. Hanna EZ, Chou SP, Grant BF. The relationship between drinking and heart disease morbidity in the United States: results from the National Health Interview Survey. Alcohol Clin Exp Res 1997;21(1):111–8.

29. Malyutina S, Bobak M, Kurilovitch S, et al. Relation between heavy and binge drinking and all-cause and cardiovascular mortality in Novosibirsk, Russia: a prospective cohort study. Lancet 2002;360(9344):1448–54.

30. Mukamal KJ, Chiuve SE, Rimm EB. Alcohol consumption and risk for coronary heart disease in men with healthy lifestyles. Arch Intern Med 2006;166(19): 2145–50.

31. Janszky I, Ljung R, Ahnve S, et al. Alcohol and long-term prognosis after a first acute myocardial infarction: the SHEEP study. Eur Heart J 2008;29(1):45–53.

32. Fiellin DA, Reid MC, O'Connor PG. Screening for alcohol problems in primary care: a systematic review. Arch Intern Med 2000;160(13):1977–89.

33. Turner RT. Skeletal response to alcohol. Alcohol Clin Exp Res 2000;24(11): 1693–701.

34. Vandenberg MK, Moxley G, Breitbach SA, et al. Gout attacks in chronic alcoholics occur at lower serum urate levels than in nonalcoholics. J Rheumatol 1994;21(4):700–4.

35. Regier DA, Farmer ME, Rae DS, et al. Comorbidity of mental disorders with alcohol and other drug abuse. Results from the Epidemiologic Catchment Area (ECA) Study. JAMA 1990;264(19):2511–8.

36. Wu LT, Kouzis AC, Leaf PJ. Influence of comorbid alcohol and psychiatric disorders on utilization of mental health services in the National Comorbidity Survey. Am J Psychiatry 1999;156(8):1230–6.

37. Sullivan LE, Fiellin DA, O'Connor PG. The prevalence and impact of alcohol problems in major depression: a systematic review. Am J Med 2005;118(4):330–41.

38. Mukamal KJ, Kawachi I, Miller M, et al. Body mass index and risk of suicide among men. Arch Intern Med 2007;167(5):468–75.

39. Cherpitel CJ, Ye Y. Alcohol-attributable fraction for injury in the U.S. general population: data from the 2005 National Alcohol Survey. J Stud Alcohol Drugs 2008; 69(4):535–8.

40. Field CA, Claassen CA, O'Keefe G. Association of alcohol use and other high-risk behaviors among trauma patients. J Trauma 2001;50(1):13–9.

41. Bell NS, Harford TC, Fuchs CH, et al. Spouse abuse and alcohol problems among white, African American, and Hispanic U.S. Army soldiers. Alcohol Clin Exp Res 2006;30(10):1721–33.

42. Hungerford DW, Pollock DA, Todd KH. Acceptability of emergency department-based screening and brief intervention for alcohol problems. Acad Emerg Med 2000;7(12):1383–92.

43. D'Amico EJ, Paddock SM, Burnam A, et al. Identification of and guidance for problem drinking by general medical providers: results from a national survey. Med Care 2005;43(3):229–36.

44. Franck J, Jayaram-Lindstrom N. Pharmacotherapy for alcohol dependence: status of current treatments. Curr Opin Neurobiol 2013;23(4):692–9.

45. Harris AH, Ellerbe L, Reeder RN, et al. Pharmacotherapy for alcohol dependence: perceived treatment barriers and action strategies among Veterans Health Administration service providers. Psychol Serv 2013;10(4):410–9.

46. Friedmann PD, Saitz R, Samet JH. Management of adults recovering from alcohol or other drug problems: relapse prevention in primary care. JAMA 1998;279(15): 1227–31.

47. DiClemente CC, Bellino LE, Neavins TM. Motivation for change and alcoholism treatment. Alcohol Res Health 1999;23(2):86–92.

48. Kaner E, Bland M, Cassidy P, et al. Effectiveness of screening and brief alcohol intervention in primary care (SIPS trial): pragmatic cluster randomised controlled trial. BMJ 2013;346:e8501.

49. Miller WR, Rollnick S. Motivational interviewing: preparing people to change addictive behavior. New York: The Guilford Press; 1991.

50. Jonas DE, Garbutt JC, Amick HR, et al. Behavioral counseling after screening for alcohol misuse in primary care: a systematic review and meta-analysis for the U.S. Preventive Services Task Force. Ann Intern Med 2012;157(9):645–54.

51. National Institute on Alcohol Abuse and Alcoholism (NIAAA). Helping patients who drink too much: a clinician's guide. Rockville (MD): NIAAA; 2007.

52. Moyer VA. Screening and behavioral counseling interventions in primary care to reduce alcohol misuse: U.S. preventive services task force recommendation statement. Ann Intern Med 2013;159(3):210–8.

53. National Alcohol Strategy Working Group. Reducing alcohol-related harm in Canada: toward a culture of moderation. Recommendations for a national alcohol strategy. Edmonton and Ottawa (Canada): Alberta Alcohol and Drug Abuse Commission; Canadian Centre on Substance Abuse and Health; 2007.

54. Sullivan LE, Tetrault JM, Braithwaite RS, et al. A meta-analysis of the efficacy of nonphysician brief interventions for unhealthy alcohol use: implications for the patient-centered medical home. Am J Addict 2011;20(4):343–56.

55. O'Donnell A, Anderson P, Newbury-Birch D, et al. The impact of brief alcohol interventions in primary healthcare: a systematic review of reviews. Alcohol 2014; 49(1):66–78.

56. Reoux JP, Miller K. Routine hospital alcohol detoxification practice compared to symptom triggered management with an Objective Withdrawal Scale (CIWA-Ar). Am J Addict 2000;9(2):135–44.

57. Fiellin DA, O'Connor PG, Holmboe ES, et al. Risk for delirium tremens in patients with alcohol withdrawal syndrome. Subst Abus 2002;23(2):83–94.

58. Pecoraro A, Ewen E, Horton T, et al. Using the AUDIT-PC to predict alcohol withdrawal in hospitalized patients. J Gen Intern Med 2014;29(1):34–40.

59. Amato L, Minozzi S, Davoli M. Efficacy and safety of pharmacological interventions for the treatment of the alcohol withdrawal syndrome. Cochrane Database Syst Rev 2011;(6):CD008537.

60. Perry EC. Inpatient management of acute alcohol withdrawal syndrome. CNS Drugs 2014;28(5):401–10.

61. National Institute for Health and Care Excellence. Alcohol use disorders: diagnosis and clinical management of alcohol-related physical complications. London: National Clinical Guideline Center; 2010.

62. Wong A, Benedict NJ, Armahizer MJ, et al. Evaluation of adjunctive ketamine to benzodiazepines for management of alcohol withdrawal syndrome. Ann Pharmacother 2015;49(1):14–9.

63. Sohraby R, Attridge RL, Hughes DW. Use of propofol-containing versus benzodi-azepine regimens for alcohol withdrawal requiring mechanical ventilation. Ann Pharmacother 2014;48(4):456–61.

64. Frazee EN, Personett HA, Leung JG, et al. Influence of dexmedetomidine therapy on the management of severe alcohol withdrawal syndrome in critically ill pa-tients. J Crit Care 2014;29(2):298–302.

65. Muzyk AJ, Kerns S, Brudney S, et al. Dexmedetomidine for the treatment of alcohol withdrawal syndrome: rationale and current status of research. CNS Drugs 2013;27(11):913–20.

66. Muncie HL Jr, Yasinian Y, Oge L. Outpatient management of alcohol withdrawal syndrome. Am Fam Physician 2013;88(9):589–95.

67. Quanbeck A, Chih MY, Isham A, et al. Mobile delivery of treatment for alcohol use disorders: a review of the literature. Alcohol Res 2014;36(1):111–22.

68. Matching alcoholism treatments to client heterogeneity: project MATCH posttreat-ment drinking outcomes. J Stud Alcohol 1997;58(1):7–29.

69. Martin GW, Rehm J. The effectiveness of psychosocial modalities in the treatment of alcohol problems in adults: a review of the evidence. Can J Psychiatry 2012; 57(6):350–8.

70. Witbrodt J, Ye Y, Bond J, et al. Alcohol and drug treatment involvement, 12-step attendance and abstinence: 9-year cross-lagged analysis of adults in an inte-grated health plan. J Subst Abuse Treat 2014;46(4):412–9.

71. Pagano ME, White WL, Kelly JF, et al. The 10-year course of Alcoholics Anony-mous participation and long-term outcomes: a follow-up study of outpatient subjects in Project MATCH. Subst Abus 2013;34(1):51–9.

72. Magura S, McKean J, Kosten S, et al. A novel application of propensity score matching to estimate Alcoholics Anonymous' effect on drinking outcomes. Drug Alcohol Depend 2013;129(1–2):54–9.

73. Zindel LR, Kranzler HR. Pharmacotherapy of alcohol use disorders: seventy-five years of progress. J Stud Alcohol Drugs Suppl 2014;75(Suppl 17):79–88.

74. Skinner MD, Lahmek P, Pham H, et al. Disulfiram efficacy in the treatment of alcohol dependence: a meta-analysis. PLoS One 2014;9(2):e87366.

75. Anton RF. Naltrexone for the management of alcohol dependence. N Engl J Med 2008;359(7):715–21.

76. Lukas SE, Lowen SB, Lindsey KP, et al. Extended-release naltrexone (XR-NTX) attenuates brain responses to alcohol cues in alcohol-dependent volunteers: a bold FMRI study. Neuroimage 2013;78:176–85.

77. Jonas DE, Amick HR, Feltner C, et al. Pharmacotherapy for adults with alcohol use disorders in outpatient settings: a systematic review and meta-analysis. JAMA 2014;311(18):1889–900.

78. Yen MH, Ko HC, Tang FI, et al. Study of hepatotoxicity of naltrexone in the treat-ment of alcoholism. Alcohol 2006;38(2):117–20.

79. Mitchell MC, Memisoglu A, Silverman BL. Hepatic safety of injectable extended-release naltrexone in patients with chronic hepatitis C and HIV infection. J Stud Alcohol Drugs 2012;73(6):991–7.

80. Higuchi S. Efficacy of acamprosate for the treatment of alcohol dependence long after recovery from withdrawal syndrome: a randomized, double-blind, placebo-controlled study conducted in Japan (Sunrise Study). J Clin Psychiatry 2015; 76(2):181–8.

81. Maisel NC, Blodgett JC, Wilbourne PL, et al. Meta-analysis of naltrexone and acamprosate for treating alcohol use disorders: when are these medications most helpful? Addiction 2013;108(2):275–93.

82. Rosenthal RN, Gage A, Perhach JL, et al. Acamprosate: safety and tolerability in the treatment of alcohol dependence. J Addict Med 2008;2(1):40–50.
83. Blodgett JC, Del Re AC, Maisel NC, et al. A meta-analysis of topiramate's effects for individuals with alcohol use disorders. Alcohol Clin Exp Res 2014;38(6): 1481–8.
84. Martinotti G, Di Nicola M, De Vita O, et al. Low-dose topiramate in alcohol dependence: a single-blind, placebo-controlled study. J Clin Psychopharmacol 2014; 34(6):709–15.
85. Laramee P, Brodtkorb TH, Rahhali N, et al. The cost-effectiveness and public health benefit of nalmefene added to psychosocial support for the reduction of alcohol consumption in alcohol-dependent patients with high/very high drinking risk levels: a Markov model. BMJ Open 2014;4(9):e005376.
86. Erwin BL, Slaton RM. Varenicline in the treatment of alcohol use disorders. Ann Pharmacother 2014;48(11):1445–55.
87. Litten RZ, Ryan ML, Fertig JB, et al. A double-blind, placebo-controlled trial assessing the efficacy of varenicline tartrate for alcohol dependence. J Addict Med 2013;7(4):277–86.
88. Guglielmo R, Martinotti G, Clerici M, et al. Pregabalin for alcohol dependence: a critical review of the literature. Adv Ther 2012;29(11):947–57.
89. Mason BJ, Quello S, Goodell V, et al. Gabapentin treatment for alcohol dependence: a randomized clinical trial. JAMA Intern Med 2014;174(1):70–7.
90. Nunes EV. Gabapentin: a new addition to the armamentarium for alcohol dependence? JAMA Intern Med 2014;174(1):78–9.

FURTHER READING

The National Institute on Alcohol Abuse and Alcoholism (NIAAA) provides guidelines for practitioners on the management of patients with alcohol-related problems. Available at: http://www.niaaa.nih.gov. The NIAAA guidelines address behavioral and social problems, as well as the medical manifestations of alcohol use.

Pathogenesis of Alcoholic Liver Disease

Winston Dunn, MD[a], Vijay H. Shah, MD[b],*

KEYWORDS

- Sterile necrosis • Corticosteroids • Alcoholic liver disease • Alcoholic hepatitis
- Intestinal permeability • Microbiome

KEY POINTS

- Alcoholic liver disease, especially alcoholic hepatitis, continues to be a major cause of liver-related morbidity and mortality.
- Alcohol and its metabolic byproducts, including acetaldehyde, contribute to liver injury.
- Liver injury leads to inflammation in alcoholic hepatitis through a classical "sterile necrosis" response.
- Enhanced gut permeability and changes in microbiome also contribute to alcoholic liver disease.
- New pathophysiology-based therapies are undergoing evaluation in patients.

SPECTRUM, RISK FACTORS, AND COMORBIDITIES

Alcoholic liver disease (ALD) includes a broad spectrum of disorders, such as simple steatosis, cirrhosis, acute alcoholic hepatitis (AH) with or without cirrhosis, and hepatocellular carcinoma (HCC) as a complication of cirrhosis. ALD can also be superimposed on other common liver diseases, including nonalcoholic liver disease (NAFLD) and hepatitis C virus (HCV) infection, accentuating their prevalence and severity. A large French study looked at 1604 biopsies on patients admitted for alcoholism or ALD and found normal liver, 14%; steatosis without fibrosis, 29%; some fibrosis ± steatosis, 20%; steatohepatitis without cirrhosis, 8%; cirrhosis total, 43%; cirrhosis and steatohepatitis, 13%.[1] An autopsy study of Missouri and Kansas motor vehicle accident victims, who were heavily intoxicated (average blood alcohol concentration, 0.22%) at the time of death, showed that the age-standardized prevalence values were 56% for hepatic steatosis, 6% for steatohepatitis, and 18% for advanced fibrosis.[2]

The authors have nothing to disclose.
[a] Gastroenterology & Hepatology, The University of Kansas Medical Center, 3901 Rainbow Boulevard, Kansas City, KS 66160, USA; [b] Gastroenterology Research Unit, Division of Gastroenterology and Hepatology, Mayo Clinic, Rochester, MN 55905, USA
* Corresponding author.
E-mail address: shah.vijay@mayo.edu

Clin Liver Dis 20 (2016) 445–456
http://dx.doi.org/10.1016/j.cld.2016.02.004
1089-3261/16/$ – see front matter © 2016 Elsevier Inc. All rights reserved.

liver.theclinics.com

Risk Factors

AH usually refers to an acute symptomatic manifestation of histologic steatohepatitis. The mouse model by Bin Gao[3] suggested that AH requires "2 hits," combining chronic heavy alcohol consumption in addition to alcohol bingeing.[4] In human studies, most subjects reported heavy alcohol use (more than 100 g/d) for 2 or more decades.[5] The patients are usually 40 to 60 years of age. Some patients report recent life events as an explanation for the escalated alcohol consumption.[6] Excessive weight is a risk factor for AH, which can result in a combination of both alcoholic and nonalcoholic steatohepatitis.[1] Patients with HCV are also more likely to develop AH and severe AH.[7]

AH is associated with female sex and an irregular (ie, binge) pattern of alcohol consumption, and cirrhosis is associated with female sex, heavy alcohol use duration greater than 15 years, and consumption greater than 200 g/d. PNPLA3 is a novel risk factor for alcoholic cirrhosis. With each additional G allele, patients are more likely to have alcoholic cirrhosis and to develop alcoholic cirrhosis with a shorter exposure to heavy drinking.[8,9]

In patients with alcoholic cirrhosis, the risk factors for the development of HCC include obesity, diabetes, active alcohol consumption, and viral hepatitis.[10–12] PNPLA3 is also a risk factor for HCC, especially in patients with ALD (and, to a lesser extent, HCV).[13]

Diagnosis

Distinguishing an alcoholic basis from a nonalcoholic basis for clinical and histologic steatohepatitis is difficult because of the unreliability of alcohol consumption history. The ALD/NAFLD Index uses the mean corpuscular volume, the aspartate aminotransferase (AST)/alanine aminotransferase (ALT) ratio, the body mass index, and gender to identify patients with an ALD component.[14] This model has been validated in hospitalized, ambulatory, and pretransplantation patients and compares favorably with other traditional and proposed biomarkers. An online calculator is readily available.[15] Acute AH should be distinguished from decompensated alcoholic cirrhosis or acute chronic liver disease. A breath Biosensor based on trimethylamine and pentane has been developed for the diagnosis of AH. Trimethylamine is generated from the diet and is metabolized in the liver, whereas pentane is a marker of oxidative stress.[16]

PATHOGENESIS
Ethanol-Mediated Liver Injury

Binge drinking and the National Institute on Alcohol Abuse and Alcoholism model
Binge-drinking AH typically occurs in patients with chronic alcohol consumption and a recent history of excessive alcohol use (**Fig. 1**). In a rodent model, ad libitum ethanol delivery through a liquid diet is only sufficient to produce liver abnormality limited to steatosis. The mouse model of chronic and binge ethanol feeding (National Institute on Alcohol Abuse and Alcoholism [NIAAA] model) developed by Gao and colleagues[17] uses 10 days of ad libitum liquid followed by acute bolus gavage. Although either phase alone causes steatosis, combining both phases causes steatohepatitis. Therefore, this model may better represent human acute AH. Similarly, effective models have also been developed by the Tsukamoto group, but require invasive intragastric feeding.[18]

Acetaldehyde

In hepatocytes, the primary pathway of ethanol metabolism is through acetaldehyde by alcohol dehydrogenase in the cytosol. Acetaldehyde is metabolized by aldehyde dehydrogenase (ALDH) in the mitochondria. Aldehyde is highly reactive and can

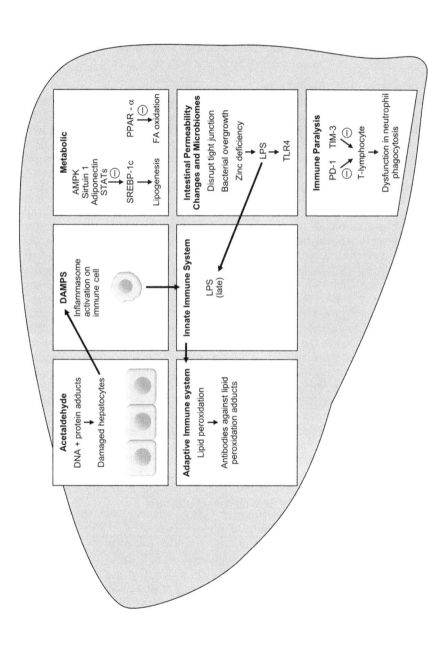

Fig. 1. Mechanisms of ALD. Alcohol contributes to liver injury through a multitude of ways as depicted. Alcohol is metabolized to acetaldehyde; both alcohol and acetaldehyde have toxic effects on hepatocytes. Damaged hepatocytes in turn release DAMPs that recruit innate and adaptive immune cells that perpetuate further liver injury. Earlier alcohol lesion of steatosis is mediated by effects of alcohol or lipogenesis and fatty acid (FA) oxidation. Alcohol also has direct effects on intestinal microbiome and gut permeability that allows bacterial products to reach liver and further stimulate immune response and liver injury. Finally, despite immune stimulation, the immune response is ineffective in combating infection, termed immune paralysis.

form various protein and DNA adducts.[19] A relative deficiency of the ALDH2 isozyme causes the accumulation of acetaldehyde. The incidence of AH is not increased because of aversion to alcohol and a lower prevalence of alcoholism. The minor pathway involves microsomal enzyme oxidation system (MEOS) and generates more reactive oxygen species, resulting in lipid peroxidation, mitochondrial gluta-thione depletion, and S-adenosylmethionine depletion. The cytochrome CYP2E1 of MEOS is induced in chronic alcoholism, further contributing to oxidative stress and liver injury.

Damage-associated molecular patterns

Alcohol metabolism leads to oxidative stress and hepatocyte death. Damaged hepa-tocytes release endogenous damage-associated molecular patterns (DAMPs), which are usually hidden from the extracellular environment. DAMPs activate cellular pattern recognition receptors, which result in sterile inflammation. Features include the pro-duction of proinflammatory cytokines, localization of immune cells to the site of injury, and assembly of a cytosolic protein complex machinery termed the "inflammasome," which convey DAMP signals into proinflammatory cytokines (eg, interleukin [IL]-1).

Metabolism

Steatosis is characterized by the accumulation of triglycerides, phospholipids, and cholesterol esters in hepatocytes. An early study attributed steatosis to the increased ratio of reduced nicotinamide adenine dinucleotide to oxidized nicotinamide adenine dinucleotide (NADH/NAD), which inhibits β-oxidation of fatty acids in mitochondria. Recent studies have indicated that alcohol consumption regulates lipid metabolism transcription factors. Alcohol stimulates lipogenesis by the upregulation of sterol reg-ulatory element-binding transcription factor 1c (SREBP-1c).[20] Alcohol can upregulate SREBP-1c directly via its metabolite acetaldehyde or indirectly via the endoplasmic reticulum stress response, adenosine, endocannabinoids, bacterial translocation, and downstream lipopolysaccharide (LPS) signaling. Alcohol also downregulates the negative regulators of SREBP-1c, including 5′ adenosine monophosphate-activated protein kinase (AMPK), Sirtuin 1 (SIRT1), adiponectin, and signal transducer and activator of transcription 3 (STAT3). Alcohol inhibits fatty acid oxidation by inhib-iting the transcriptional activity and DNA-binding ability of peroxisome proliferator-activated receptor α (PPAR-α).[21] Alcohol can downregulate PPAR-α directly via its metabolite acetaldehyde or indirectly via the cytochrome P450 2E1-derived oxidative stress, adenosine, downregulation of adiponectin, and zinc deficiency. Alcohol con-sumption can also indirectly modify many factors, including hypoxia-inducible fac-tor-1,[22] C3,[23] C1qa, PKCϵ (Protein kinase C epsilon),[24] and inducible nitric oxide synthase,[25] which contribute to the development of steatosis.

Inflammatory Immune Response to Injury

Innate immune system

Innate immune signaling is involved in the early stage of ALD with simple steatosis even before the onset of inflammation. Endoplasmic reticulum stress activates inter-feron regulatory factor 3 (IRF3) via the adaptor molecule STRING. IRF3 is phosphory-lated (activated) with a single exposure to alcohol, preceding the development of inflammation.[26] Hepatocyte-specific IRF3 is required for the intrinsic (mitochondrial) apoptosis pathway, whereas Kupffer cell IRF3 deficiency provides only marginal dam-age from liver damage.[27]

Bacterial overload and increased gut permeability lead to an increased load of bacteria-derived LPS to the portal circulation and liver. LPS interacts with toll-like receptor 4 (TLR4) on Kupffer cells, activating the Toll/interleukin-1 receptor (TIR)-domain-containing adapter-inducing interferon-β/IRF-3 signaling pathway, leading to the production of proinflammatory cytokines (ie, tumor necrosis factor-α [TNF-α], IL-1, and IL-17). Alcohol also activates the complement system (C3, C4). The interaction between complement and Kupffer cells leads to proinflammatory cytokines (TNF-α) as well as hepatoprotective (IL-6) and cytoprotective (IL-10) cytokines. TNF-α, palmitic acid, the downregulation of proteasome functions, and IL-17 cause hepatocytes (IL-8, CXCL1, and IL-17) and hepatic stellate cells (HSCs [IL-8 and CXCL1]) to produce chemokines for neutrophil recruitment.

Adaptive immunity
Chronic alcohol leads to lipid peroxidation. Lipid peroxidation products, such as malondialdehyde and 4-hydroxynonenal, can form protein adducts and serve as antigens to activate adaptive immunity. Antibodies against lipid peroxidation adducts and increased numbers of T cells in liver inflammation have been reported.[21]

Immune paralysis
The leading cause of death in AH is overwhelming bacterial infection, leading to multiorgan failure. Paradoxically, immune activity is heightened with inflammation. Programmed cell death protein 1 (PD-1) and T-cell immunoglobulin and mucin protein 3 (TIM-3) are inhibitory receptors on T lymphocytes expressed during chronic inflammation and can lead to immune exhaustion. PD-1 and TIM-3 are overexpressed in AH patients, more so than stable advanced alcoholic cirrhosis patients. The associated dysfunction in neutrophil phagocytosis and oxidative burst in response to *Escherichia coli* stimulation (in vitro) can be reversed by antibodies against PD-1 and TIM-3.[28]

Intestinal Permeability Changes and Microbiome

ALD is associated with bacterial overgrowth and a lower proportion of Bacteroidaceae and probiotic bacteria such as *Lactobacillus*. Causes include small intestinal dysmotility and alterations in bile acid pool.[29] Ethanol disrupts intestinal tight junction integrity.[30] Patients with chronic alcohol abuse with or without ALD have a "leaky gut," as evidenced by a higher level of plasma endotoxin than that in healthy control subjects.[31] In animal models, protection from bacterial overgrowth via genetic mutation[32] or antibiotics,[33] or the expression of nonfunctional TLR4 (LPS receptor),[34] can all attenuate alcohol-induced liver injury.

Zinc

Zinc deficiency is common in ALD. Animal models have demonstrated that zinc deficiency attenuates alcohol-induced liver injury through various mechanisms, but most importantly, zinc deficiency impairs the intestinal barrier,[35] leading to endotoxin-induced cytokine production. In mouse models, ethanol exposure reduces plasma leptin level,[36] stimulates white adipose tissue lipolysis,[37,38] and inhibits hepatic fatty acid oxidation. Dietary zinc deficiency worsens the alcohol-induced decline of plasma leptin and impairs hepatic fatty acid oxidation.[39] Zinc also has antioxidant properties. Dietary zinc deficiency can also lead to downregulation of antioxidant enzymes, including superoxide dismutase 1.[39]

Impaired Regeneration

Usually, liver damage induces mature hepatocytes to proliferate and replace damaged tissue. Given massive or chronic liver damage that is beyond the proliferative capacity of hepatocytes, progenitor cells proliferate to produce a ductular reaction. KRT7 is a marker of ductular reaction in liver disease, and it is typically expressed in liver progenitor cells. Prominin-1 (PROM1) is a marker of progenitor cells from the liver and is considered a marker for hepatic cancer stem cells. Both markers, as measured by real-time PCR in hepatic gene expression analysis, are associated with short-term mortality in AH. In a cohort of 59 patients with biopsy, KRT7, PROM1, model for end-stage liver disease (MELD) score, and ABIC (Age, serum Bilirubin, INR [international normalized ratio], and serum Creatinine) score were independent predictors for 90-day mortality.[36] In a study that examined explants from AH salvage transplants, a near absence of hepatocyte proliferation was noted.[26] Hepatic progenitor cells were increased, but all expressed laminin (extracellular matrix protein favoring cholangiocyte differentiation) and were therefore inefficient at yielding mature hepatocytes.

Epigenetics and MicroRNAs

MicroRNAs (miRNAs) are short noncoding RNAs that are an average of only 22 nucleotides long. They control the expression of genes involved in cell growth, differentiation, and apoptosis and are thought to be involved in the pathogenesis of liver disease, particularly cancer. The level of plasma miRNA-155 correlates with liver inflammation induced by alcohol and may be used potentially as a biomarker.[40] Short-term alcohol exposure upregulates miRNA-212 in intestinal epithelial cells, downregulating zonula occludens-1 protein, a protein that regulates intestinal permeability. Alcohol upregulates miRNA-217, which induces lipid synthesis and reduces fatty acid oxidation in the liver via inhibiting the AMPK and SIRT1 pathways.[30] Chronic alcohol also decreases the expression of miRNA 196a and c, which are involved in early regeneration.[41] The expression of liver miRNAs has also been shown to be significantly altered in alcohol-fed mice, but the functions of these miRNAs in the pathogenesis of ALD are not clear.

Protective Mechanisms

Autophagy

Selective autophagy is a protective mechanism for removing lipid droplets, protein aggregates, and damaged organelles from hepatocytes.[42] In a mouse model, alcohol may activate autophagy in hepatocytes to remove lipid droplets and damaged mitochondria, and therefore, attenuate alcohol-induced steatosis and liver injury. Lipophagy, the autophagy of alcohol-induced lipid droplets, has also been identified.[43] The induction of autophagy can potentially be an approach for treating alcohol-induced liver injury.[44] Autophagy in HSCs, on the other hand, promotes liver fibrosis by using free fatty acids as an energy source.[45]

Forkhead box O3

Forkhead Box O3 (FOXO3) plays an important role in the protection against alcohol-induced liver injury through the regulation of autophagy,[46] antioxidants,[47] and pro-apoptosis-related gene expression. FOXO3 is regulated by posttranscriptional modifications, including phosphorylation by protein kinase B (Akt) and deacetylation by Sirt1. The dephosphorylated and deacetylated forms are retained in the nucleus and can bind to promoters of target genes. Alcohol can potentially affect FOXO3 at multiple levels. Alcohol inhibits Akt phosphorylation and increases the nuclear retention of FOXO3. Alcohol metabolism increases the NADH/NAD ratio, which decreases Sirt1-mediated deacetylation. Resveratrol, a polyphenol antioxidant found in wine, is also an SIRT1 agonist. Combining alcohol and resveratrol (mouse model) can overcome the alcohol-induced Sirt1 inhibition and further increase autophagy and antioxidant-related gene expression.

The FOXO3 mechanism may also explain why patients with HCV do poorly with alcohol abuse. Either alcohol or HCV alone increases FOXO3 nuclear retention, but the combination has the opposite effect.[47] HCV promotes c-Jun N-terminal kinase

(JNK) phosphorylation at Ser574 on FOXO3, which promotes nuclear retention. Alcohol inhibits arginine-methylation of FOXO3, which promotes nuclear export and degradation of the phosphorylated form of JNK.[48]

Hepatocellular Carcinoma Development in Alcoholic Liver Disease

The general mechanism for the development of HCC includes (i) limitation of the regenerative reserve and induction of chromosomal instability by telomeres, (ii) cancer induction by the loss of replicative competition due to impaired hepatocyte proliferation, (iii) an altered microenvironment promoting tumor cell proliferation, and (iv) the loss of cell cycle check point, including resistance to apoptosis and activation of oncogenic pathways. A few of these mechanisms are specific to ALD.[49] Acetaldehyde itself is a carcinogen with mutagenic properties. Alcohol also has an immunosuppressive effect. In HCV-infected patients, alcohol can upregulate cancer stem cells.[50]

CURRENT THERAPIES AND FUTURE APPROACHES

For more information on specific therapies for AH, please see Paulina K. Phillips, Michael R. Lucey: Acute Alcoholic Hepatitis – Therapy and Srinivasan Dasarathy: Nutrition and Alcoholic Liver Disease- Effects of Alcoholism on Nutrition, Effects of Nutrition on ALD and Nutritional Therapies for ALD, in this issue. A few potential therapies that relate to the molecular pathogenesis of ALD are addressed.

S-Adenosylmethionine

Alcohol affects multiple steps in methionine metabolism. S-adenosylmethionine (SAM) is the substrate for the methylation reaction. After donating the methyl group, SAM is converted to S-adenosylhomocysteine (SAH). SAM can be regenerated via a folate-dependent or folate-independent pathway that uses betaine as a substrate. It has been hypothesized that chronic alcohol consumption decreases SAM to the SAH level, leading to mitochondrial damage and endoplasmic reticulum stress. In human studies, the treatment of ALD patients with SAM or placebo has not resulted in any difference in histopathology, AST, ALT, or bilirubin level.[51,52]

Microbiome, Lipopolysaccharide, and the Gut Barrier

Selective intestinal decontamination has been shown to improve liver hemodynamics in decompensated alcoholic cirrhosis.[53] Rifaximin has been shown to improve thrombocytopenia (a marker of portal hypertension) and MELD in alcoholic cirrhosis through the reduction of endotoxemia.[54] Probiotics have been shown to improve neutrophil function, cytokine response, and liver function. These previous studies have conceptually shown the role of microbiome/LPS/gut barrier in ALD, leading to 3 National Institutes of Health (NIH) consortia studies. The first study will focus on the anti-LPS antibody in combination with corticosteroid; the second will study probiotics, and the third will study the efficacy of zinc in restoring the integrity of the gut barrier.

Interleukin-1 Antagonist

Kupffer cells bear the receptor for DAMPs and LPS and activate the innate immune system via several cytokines, including TNF-α, IL-6, and IL-1β. The IL1 receptor antagonist anakinra will be tested in the NIH consortium.[55]

Inhibition of Apoptosis

Although studies on TNF-α inhibition have failed, the NIH consortium will focus on caspase inhibition in hepatocytes; caspase is a death induction molecule downstream of

TNF-α signaling. Caspase inhibition with emricasan may circumvent the immunosuppression and regeneration-blocking effect of TNF-α blockade and may dampen the innate immune system activation cascade through sterile necrosis and DAMPs release. A phase II clinical trial in nonalcoholic steatohepatitis (NASH) showed that caspase inhibition improved liver enzyme activity.[56]

Farnesoid X Receptor

Farnesoid X receptor (FXR) engages in a negative feedback loop for bile acid homeostasis. It negatively regulates lipogenesis through the SREBP1 and liver X receptor/SHP (small heterodimer partner) axis and positively regulates fatty acid oxidation through PPARα, potentially counteracting the steatosis pathophysiology in NASH and ALD. More importantly, FXR activation may downregulate HSC activation and, therefore, has antifibrotic properties.[57] Currently, FXR agonist studies are still underway for both NASH and alcoholic steatohepatitis.

Interleukin-22

IL-22[58] is produced by Th17 cells and natural killer cells. The biological effect is mediated mainly via activation of the STAT3 signaling pathway through the binding of IL-22R1 and IL-10R2. In a murine model of chronic-binge alcohol feeding, treatment with IL-22 recombinant protein activates hepatic STAT3 and ameliorates alcoholic fatty liver, liver injury, and hepatic oxidative stress. In patients with AH, expression of IL-22R1 is upregulated, whereas IL-22 is undetectable, suggesting that IL-22 treatment could be a potential therapeutic option.

Osteopontin

Osteopontin is a chemoattractant for polymorphonuclear leukocytes and promotes fibrosis in NASH. The role of osteopontin has been controversial in ALD depending on the experimental model. Lazaro and colleagues[59] used the NIAAA model of acute AH superimposed on a background of severe steatosis and demonstrated that osteopontin deficiency does not prevent, but rather promotes, AH, suggesting a potential therapeutic target.

Cannabinoid

Cannabinoid receptor type 1 (CB1) is a promoter of fibrosis, whereas Cannabinoid receptor type 2 (CB2) is an inhibitor.[60] In response to alcohol feeding, steatosis and fibrogenesis are increased in CB2 receptor-deficient mice and decreased in CB1 receptor knockouts.[61] Rimonabant is a CB1 antagonist used in Europe for the treatment of obesity and metabolic syndrome, before it was withdrawn from the market for its adverse effect of depression. Nonpsychoactive cannabinoids are currently being developed.[62]

REFERENCES

1. Naveau S, Giraud V, Borotto E, et al. Excess weight risk factor for alcoholic liver disease. Hepatology 1997;25(1):108–11.
2. Dunn W, Zeng Z, O'Neil M, et al. The interaction of rs738409, obesity, and alcohol: a population-based autopsy study. Am J Gastroenterol 2012;107(11):1668–74.
3. Bertola A, Mathews S, Ki SH, et al. Mouse model of chronic and binge ethanol feeding (the NIAAA model). Nat Protoc 2013;8(3):627–37.
4. Deng QG, She H, Cheng JH, et al. Steatohepatitis induced by intragastric overfeeding in mice. Hepatology 2005;42(4):905–14.

5. Cohen SM, Ahn J. Review article: the diagnosis and management of alcoholic hepatitis. Aliment Pharmacol Ther 2009;30(1):3–13.
6. Choi G, Runyon BA. Alcoholic hepatitis: a clinician's guide. Clin Liver Dis 2012; 16(2):371–85.
7. Punzalan CS, Bukong TN, Szabo G. Alcoholic hepatitis and HCV interactions in the modulation of liver disease. J Viral Hepat 2015;22(10):769–76.
8. Tian C, Stokowski RP, Kershenobich D, et al. Variant in PNPLA3 is associated with alcoholic liver disease. Nat Genet 2010;42(1):21–3.
9. Burza MA, Molinaro A, Attilia ML, et al. PNPLA3 I148M (rs738409) genetic variant and age at onset of at-risk alcohol consumption are independent risk factors for alcoholic cirrhosis. Liver Int 2014;34(4):514–20.
10. Saunders D, Seidel D, Allison M, et al. Systematic review: the association between obesity and hepatocellular carcinoma—epidemiological evidence. Aliment Pharmacol Ther 2010;31(10):1051–63.
11. Loomba R, Yang HI, Su J, et al. Synergism between obesity and alcohol in increasing the risk of hepatocellular carcinoma: a prospective cohort study. Am J Epidemiol 2013;177(4):333–42.
12. Donato F, Tagger A, Gelatti U, et al. Alcohol and hepatocellular carcinoma: the effect of lifetime intake and hepatitis virus infections in men and women. Am J Epidemiol 2002;155(4):323–31.
13. Trepo E, Nahon P, Bontempi G, et al. Association between the PNPLA3 (rs738409 C>G) variant and hepatocellular carcinoma: evidence from a meta-analysis of individual participant data. Hepatology 2014;59(6):2170–7.
14. Dunn W, Angulo P, Sanderson S, et al. Utility of a new model to diagnose an alcohol basis for steatohepatitis. Gastroenterology 2006;131(4):1057–63.
15. Available at: http://www.mayoclinic.org/medical-professionals/model-end-stage-liver-disease/alcoholic-liver-disease-nonalcoholic-fatty-liver-disease-index. Accessed March 17, 2016.
16. Hanouneh IA, Zein NN, Cikach F, et al. The breathprints in patients with liver disease identify novel breath biomarkers in alcoholic hepatitis. Clin Gastroenterol Hepatol 2014;12(3):516–23.
17. Arteel GE. Build a better mouse model, and the world will beat a path to your door. Hepatology 2013;58(5):1526–8.
18. Tsukamoto H, French SW, Reidelberger RD, et al. Cyclical pattern of blood alcohol levels during continuous intragastric ethanol infusion in rats. Alcohol Clin Exp Res 1985;9(1):31–7.
19. Setshedi M, Wands JR, Monte SM. Acetaldehyde adducts in alcoholic liver disease. Oxid Med Cell Longev 2010;3(3):178–85.
20. Ji C, Chan C, Kaplowitz N. Predominant role of sterol response element binding proteins (SREBP) lipogenic pathways in hepatic steatosis in the murine intragastric ethanol feeding model. J Hepatol 2006;45(5):717–24.
21. Li HH, Tyburski JB, Wang YW, et al. Modulation of fatty acid and bile acid metabolism by peroxisome proliferator-activated receptor alpha protects against alcoholic liver disease. Alcohol Clin Exp Res 2014;38(6):1520–31.
22. Nath B, Levin I, Csak T, et al. Hepatocyte-specific hypoxia-inducible factor-1alpha is a determinant of lipid accumulation and liver injury in alcohol-induced steatosis in mice. Hepatology 2011;53(5):1526–37.
23. Pritchard MT, McMullen MR, Stavitsky AB, et al. Differential contributions of C3, C5, and decay-accelerating factor to ethanol-induced fatty liver in mice. Gastroenterology 2007;132(3):1117–26.

24. Kaiser JP, Beier JI, Zhang J, et al. PKCepsilon plays a causal role in acute ethanol-induced steatosis. Arch Biochem Biophys 2009;482(1–2):104–11.

25. McKim SE, Gabele E, Isayama F, et al. Inducible nitric oxide synthase is required in alcohol-induced liver injury: studies with knockout mice. Gastroenterology 2003;125(6):1834–44.

26. Petrasek J, Iracheta-Vellve A, Csak T, et al. STING-IRF3 pathway links endoplasmic reticulum stress with hepatocyte apoptosis in early alcoholic liver disease. Proc Natl Acad Sci U S A 2013;110(41):16544–9.

27. Petrasek J, Dolganiuc A, Csak T, et al. Interferon regulatory factor 3 and type I interferons are protective in alcoholic liver injury in mice by way of crosstalk of parenchymal and myeloid cells. Hepatology 2011;53(2):649–60.

28. Markwick LJ, Riva A, Ryan JM, et al. Blockade of PD1 and TIM3 restores innate and adaptive immunity in patients with acute alcoholic hepatitis. Gastroenterology 2015;148(3):590–602.e510.

29. Kakiyama G, Pandak WM, Gillevet PM, et al. Modulation of the fecal bile acid profile by gut microbiota in cirrhosis. J Hepatol 2013;58(5):949–55.

30. Yin H, Hu M, Zhang R, et al. MicroRNA-217 promotes ethanol-induced fat accumulation in hepatocytes by down-regulating SIRT1. J Biol Chem 2012;287(13): 9817–26.

31. Elamin EE, Masclee AA, Dekker J, et al. Ethanol metabolism and its effects on the intestinal epithelial barrier. Nutr Rev 2013;71(7):483–99.

32. Parlesak A, Schafer C, Schutz T, et al. Increased intestinal permeability to macromolecules and endotoxemia in patients with chronic alcohol abuse in different stages of alcohol-induced liver disease. J Hepatol 2000;32(5):742–7.

33. Adachi Y, Moore LE, Bradford BU, et al. Antibiotics prevent liver injury in rats following long-term exposure to ethanol. Gastroenterology 1995;108(1):218–24.

34. Uesugi T, Froh M, Arteel GE, et al. Toll-like receptor 4 is involved in the mechanism of early alcohol-induced liver injury in mice. Hepatology 2001;34(1):101–8.

35. Zhong W, McClain CJ, Cave M, et al. The role of zinc deficiency in alcohol-induced intestinal barrier dysfunction. Am J Physiol Gastrointest Liver Physiol 2010;298(5):G625–33.

36. Tan X, Sun X, Li Q, et al. Leptin deficiency contributes to the pathogenesis of alcoholic fatty liver disease in mice. Am J Pathol 2012;181(4):1279–86.

37. Zhong W, Zhao Y, Tang Y, et al. Chronic alcohol exposure stimulates adipose tissue lipolysis in mice: role of reverse triglyceride transport in the pathogenesis of alcoholic steatosis. Am J Pathol 2012;180(3):998–1007.

38. Wei X, Shi X, Zhong W, et al. Chronic alcohol exposure disturbs lipid homeostasis at the adipose tissue-liver axis in mice: analysis of triacylglycerols using high-resolution mass spectrometry in combination with in vivo metabolite deuterium labeling. PLoS One 2013;8(2):e55382.

39. Zhong W, Zhao Y, Sun X, et al. Dietary zinc deficiency exaggerates ethanol-induced liver injury in mice: involvement of intrahepatic and extrahepatic factors. PLoS One 2013;8(10):e76522.

40. Bala S, Petrasek J, Mundkur S, et al. Circulating microRNAs in exosomes indicate hepatocyte injury and inflammation in alcoholic, drug-induced, and inflammatory liver diseases. Hepatology 2012;56(5):1946–57.

41. Dippold RP, Vadigepalli R, Gonye GE, et al. Chronic ethanol feeding alters miRNA expression dynamics during liver regeneration. Alcohol Clin Exp Res 2013; 37(Suppl 1):E59–69.

42. Czaja MJ, Ding WX, Donohue TM Jr, et al. Functions of autophagy in normal and diseased liver. Autophagy 2013;9(8):1131–58.

43. Ronis MJ, Mercer KE, Gannon B, et al. Increased 4-hydroxynonenal protein adducts in male GSTA4-4/PPAR-alpha double knockout mice enhance injury during early stages of alcoholic liver disease. Am J Physiol Gastrointest Liver Physiol 2015;308(5):G403–15.
44. Ding WX. Induction of autophagy, a promising approach for treating liver injury. Hepatology 2014;59(1):340–3.
45. Hernandez-Gea V, Ghiassi-Nejad Z, Rozenfeld R, et al. Autophagy releases lipid that promotes fibrogenesis by activated hepatic stellate cells in mice and in human tissues. Gastroenterology 2012;142(4):938–46.
46. Ni HM, Du K, You M, et al. Critical role of FoxO3a in alcohol-induced autophagy and hepatotoxicity. Am J Pathol 2013;183(6):1815–25.
47. Tumurbaatar B, Tikhanovich I, Li Z, et al. Hepatitis C and alcohol exacerbate liver injury by suppression of FOXO3. Am J Pathol 2013;183(6):1803–14.
48. Tikhanovich I, Kuravi S, Campbell RV, et al. Regulation of FOXO3 by phosphorylation and methylation in hepatitis C virus infection and alcohol exposure. Hepatology 2014;59(1):58–70.
49. McKillop IH, Schrum LW. Role of alcohol in liver carcinogenesis. Semin Liver Dis 2009;29(2):222–32.
50. Machida K, Tsukamoto H, Mkrtchyan H, et al. Toll-like receptor 4 mediates synergism between alcohol and HCV in hepatic oncogenesis involving stem cell marker Nanog. Proc Natl Acad Sci U S A 2009;106(5):1548–53.
51. Le MD, Enbom E, Traum PK, et al. Alcoholic liver disease patients treated with S-adenosyl-L-methionine: an in-depth look at liver morphologic data comparing pre and post treatment liver biopsies. Exp Mol Pathol 2013;95(2):187–91.
52. Medici V, Virata MC, Peerson JM, et al. S-adenosyl-L-methionine treatment for alcoholic liver disease: a double-blinded, randomized, placebo-controlled trial. Alcohol Clin Exp Res 2011;35(11):1960–5.
53. Seo YS, Shah VH. The role of gut-liver axis in the pathogenesis of liver cirrhosis and portal hypertension. Clin Mol Hepatol 2012;18(4):337–46.
54. Kalambokis GN, Mouzaki A, Rodi M, et al. Rifaximin improves thrombocytopenia in patients with alcoholic cirrhosis in association with reduction of endotoxaemia. Liver Int 2012;32(3):467–75.
55. Petrasek J, Bala S, Csak T, et al. IL-1 receptor antagonist ameliorates inflammasome-dependent alcoholic steatohepatitis in mice. J Clin Invest 2012; 122(10):3476–89.
56. Ratziu V, Sheikh MY, Sanyal AJ, et al. A phase 2, randomized, double-blind, placebo-controlled study of GS-9450 in subjects with nonalcoholic steatohepatitis. Hepatology 2012;55(2):419–28.
57. Verbeke L, Farre R, Trebicka J, et al. Obeticholic acid, a farnesoid X receptor agonist, improves portal hypertension by two distinct pathways in cirrhotic rats. Hepatology 2014;59(6):2286–98.
58. Ki SH, Park O, Zheng M, et al. Interleukin-22 treatment ameliorates alcoholic liver injury in a murine model of chronic-binge ethanol feeding: role of signal transducer and activator of transcription 3. Hepatology 2010;52(4):1291–300.
59. Lazaro R, Wu R, Lee S, et al. Osteopontin deficiency does not prevent but promotes alcoholic neutrophilic hepatitis in mice. Hepatology 2015;61(1): 129–40.
60. Basu PP, Aloysius MM, Shah NJ, et al. Review article: the endocannabinoid system in liver disease, a potential therapeutic target. Aliment Pharmacol Ther 2014; 39(8):790–801.

61. Trebicka J, Racz I, Siegmund SV, et al. Role of cannabinoid receptors in alcoholic hepatic injury: steatosis and fibrogenesis are increased in CB2 receptor-deficient mice and decreased in CB1 receptor knockouts. Liver Int 2011;31(6):860–70.

62. Silvestri C, Paris D, Martella A, et al. Two non-psychoactive cannabinoids reduce intracellular lipid levels and inhibit hepatosteatosis. J Hepatol 2015;62(6): 1382–90.

Diagnosis of Alcoholic Liver Disease

Key Foundations and New Developments

Ryan E. Childers, MD[a], Joseph Ahn, MD, MS[b],*

KEYWORDS

- Alcoholic liver disease • Alcoholic hepatitis • Alcoholic fatty liver disease
- Chronic alcoholic liver disease • Cirrhosis

KEY POINTS

- There are three main clinical entities encompassing alcoholic liver disease (alcoholic fatty liver disease, alcoholic hepatitis, and chronic alcoholic liver disease), and each is increasing in prevalence and represents a growing economic burden in health care.
- The patient history and a detailed physical examination remain the cornerstones of diagnosing alcoholic liver disease.
- Clinicians should understand the value and relevance of routine laboratory indices, imaging studies, and histopathology, and how to apply these tools on a case-by-case basis in patients with alcoholic liver disease.
- Novel biomarkers, scoring systems, and imaging modalities are improving the ability to diagnose and manage alcoholic liver disease, but for most practicing clinicians, these are evolving tools that are not ready for routine implementation.
- Liver biopsy has become sparingly used in the diagnosis of alcoholic liver disease, but retains importance in specific scenarios.

INTRODUCTION

Alcoholic liver disease (ALD) encompasses a spectrum of liver injury patterns caused by the use and abuse of alcohol.[1,2] Generally, there are three main clinical entities encompassing ALD. The first is alcoholic fatty liver disease (AFLD), which can occur with or without evidence of steatohepatitis. The second is acute alcoholic hepatitis (AH), which is a clinical syndrome representing an acute pattern of liver injury often

Disclosure Statement: The authors have nothing to disclose.
[a] Division of Gastroenterology, Department of Medicine, Oregon Health and Science University, 3181 Southwest Sam Jackson Park Road, Mailcode L-461, Portland, OR 97239, USA;
[b] Division of Gastroenterology, Department of Medicine, Oregon Health and Science University, 3181 Southwest Sam Jackson Park Road, Portland, OR 97239, USA
* Corresponding author.
E-mail address: ahnj@ohsu.edu

overlying chronic injury from prolonged alcohol use. The third is chronic ALD, caused by long-standing alcohol use, often with underlying hepatic fibrosis or cirrhosis. Each of these three clinical entities is becoming more prevalent in the United States as rates of alcohol consumption continue to rise.[3,4]

The approach to the diagnosis of ALD continues to rely heavily on a careful history and physical examination, but also requires an understanding of routine laboratory indices, imaging studies, and histopathology. Novel serum markers and other diagnostic tools are opening new frontiers in the diagnosis of ALD, but are not ready for routine implementation.

RISK FACTORS

Understanding of the risk factors for ALD has improved during the last 20 years, but remains imperfect. It is now established that ALD is more common in patients aged 40 to 50 years old, obese patients, and in women (secondary to decreased gastric mucosal alcohol dehydrogenase and therefore increased hepatic metabolism).[5] The type of alcohol seems less important than the amount, but predicting the absolute amount of alcohol that leads to ALD in any given patient remains challenging. Updated U.S. guidelines now suggest lower thresholds for men (>210 g weekly or >30 g daily) and women (>140 g weekly or >20 g daily).[6] Of note, European guidelines continue to advocate higher thresholds (>60 g daily for men, >30 g daily for women) for risk in developing ALD.[7]

Although "social drinking," defined as a maximum of 30 g of alcohol daily (one standard drink contains roughly 14 g of alcohol), can predispose an individual to ALD, most individuals who consume greater than this amount are still unlikely to develop ALD.[8,9] Among patients who consume greater than 120 g of alcohol daily, there is as little as a 13% risk of developing ALD, and only 2.2% of such patients in a representative cohort developed cirrhosis.[10] Risks also seem to vary based on ethnicity, with white Hispanic men and women at higher risk of cirrhosis and mortality from ALD than other populations.[11] Furthermore, although increased alcohol consumption seems to increase the risk of ALD development, this correlation is not linear. Some cases of ALD may have an accelerated progression because of the impact of concomitant liver diseases, such as chronic viral hepatitis and non-AFLD.[12]

HISTORY

Establishing a diagnosis of ALD requires a thorough history from the patient. Historical details provided by the patient remain more sensitive and less expensive than biochemical tests in general outpatient practice settings, and allow initiation of the physician-patient relationship.[13] There are many validated tools that are helpful in primary care settings to identify patients who have or are at risk of having alcoholism, including the CAGE, MAST, AUDIT-C, or single-item screening tests. For more information on these tools, please see Pierre M. Gholam: Prognosis and Prognostic Scoring Models for Alcoholic Liver Disease and Acute Alcoholic Hepatitis, in this issue. The U.S. Preventive Services Task Force recommends the use of the AUDIT-C or single-item screening tests.[14] However, in evaluating for ALD (as opposed to alcoholism alone), it is important to elicit further detail of alcohol use beyond what is contained in these screening tools, and to inquire about risk factors for other types of liver disease.

Having a frank discussion with patients about their alcohol use is difficult. Patients, especially young men and middle-aged women, may underestimate by 40% to 50% the amount of alcohol they consume.[15] Patients may also purposefully underreport their actual alcohol consumption because of shame or embarrassment.[16] It is therefore important for the clinician to destigmatize alcohol use by conveying to the patient that clinical facts necessary to an accurate diagnosis and treatment plan, and not social judgment, are the reasons for detailed questions regarding alcohol consumption. Family members, if available for interview, may be a valuable source of further information regarding a patient's alcohol use.

In general, clinicians should understand the length of time a patient has used alcohol, the peak amount of daily alcohol use, the current daily average amount of alcohol consumption, the pattern of use, the ramifications of use, and prior attempts to quit or cut back (**Table 1**).

A family history of alcoholism is helpful to make the diagnosis of ALD because it confers an increased risk of alcohol use beginning at a younger age and increased severity of alcoholism, with a recent multiple regression analysis showing that having three or more alcoholic family members independently predicts more severe alcoholism (>480 g of alcohol weekly) for a given patient.[17] A family history of alcoholism in a patient with ALD may also predict a higher rate of eventual relapse.[18] These details may potentially impact management of patients with ALD by signaling a need for a

Table 1 Suggested questions when evaluating for alcoholic liver disease	
General Topics	**Specific Questions**
History of use, pattern of use	1. How old were you when you started using alcohol? 2. What types of alcohol did you consume in the past, and what types do you regularly consume now? 3. How much alcohol do you consume daily, or weekly? 4. How do you use alcohol? Do you use it after work, on weekends, in the morning, and/or before bed? 5. If you used to consume more alcohol in the past, can you estimate the average highest amount you used, and for how long you used this higher amount? 6. How often do you binge drink (>5 drinks for men or >4 drinks for women at one time)?[a] 7. When was your last drink?
Medical, social, and economic ramifications of use	1. How has your health been affected by your alcohol use? 2. Has your alcohol use ever affected your career or employment? 3. Have you ever had a DUI citation (driving under the influence)? 4. Have you ever been arrested or had other citations related to your alcohol use? 5. Has your alcohol use ever affected your relationships with friends and family? 6. Does your spouse/partner/family member consume alcohol with you?
Previous attempts to quit, cut back, or rehabilitate	1. Have you ever tried to cut back or quit alcohol on your own, and if so, were you successful? 2. What was the longest period of time you were abstinent? 3. Have you ever been told by family or friends that you should seek help for your alcohol use? 4. Have you ever attended an alcohol rehabilitation or detoxification program? 5. Do you attend or have you ever attended Alcoholics Anonymous?

[a] National Institute of Alcohol Abuse and Alcoholism definition of binge drinking.

more intensive approach to relapse risk reduction and in risk stratifying patients who are being considered for liver transplant candidacy.

The pursuit of a diagnosis of ALD should not preclude consideration of alternative or concomitant diagnoses, including drug-induced liver injury, viral hepatitis, autoimmune hepatitis, and genetic or metabolic liver diseases, notably hemochromatosis. Patients should be asked about recent or current illicit drug use, over-the-counter medication use (eg, acetaminophen), and dietary or herbal supplements.[2] Focus should also be given to excluding other syndromes that can cause or exacerbate liver injury, such as congestive heart failure, obesity, inflammatory bowel disease, celiac disease, and thyroid disease.

The diagnosis of AH, which unlike AFLD or chronic ALD is more often made in the inpatient setting, should involve further exploration of triggers or causes of the acute illness, which may have resulted in increased alcohol use before presentation. Paradoxically, patients may report a reduced desire to drink alcohol or complete cessation of alcohol weeks before presentation, and may recognize that their acute symptoms are caused by alcohol use. Patients should be asked about recent life stressors, including death of family or friends, job loss, and divorce.[16] A history of trauma, lacerations, or recent falls may be suggestive of recent heavy alcohol use.[8] Patients in private health care systems or patients from higher socioeconomic backgrounds may not be questioned as carefully.[16] Clinicians should be aware of this potential for bias to maintain an accurate and rigorous diagnostic approach to ALD.

SYMPTOMS AND PHYSICAL EXAMINATION

AFLD (simple steatosis), AH, and chronic ALD can manifest clinically as specific entities, with symptoms and physical examination findings defined by and correlating with the degree and onset time of liver injury.[19] However, overlap of symptoms and physical examination signs may exist, because some patients may have more than one subset of ALD (especially AH and chronic ALD). Certain features of ALD are more specific to these subset entities (discussed next).

AFLD is generally an asymptomatic condition. The physical examination is usually unremarkable, although mild hepatomegaly may be appreciated. Hepatomegaly is inferred by palpating or percussing the liver span, but this has been shown to poorly correlate with actual liver volume.[20] Furthermore, examining the liver may be difficult not only in obese patients but in normal-weight individuals, and these findings are prone to significant interobserver variability.[21] At times, nonhepatic symptoms of alcoholism can aid in the diagnosis of AFLD and ALD in general: numbness (peripheral neuropathy), dyspnea or fatigue (cardiomyopathy), weight loss and diarrhea (pancreatic insufficiency), and psychiatric or neurologic dysfunction.

Patients with AH may occasionally be asymptomatic, but typical symptoms include jaundice, malaise, fatigue, anorexia, and fever. Jaundice usually develops within 3 months of onset of injury, and is frequently reported by the patient or family members. On physical examination, the most common finding is tender hepatomegaly with or without right upper quadrant abdominal pain, which is thought to be secondary to cellular swelling and intrahepatic fatty deposition.[22] Fever can be noted, sometimes as high as 104°F, and should always prompt exclusion of an infectious cause.[23] Sarcopenia in proximal muscle groups and decreased grip strength, both of which suggest advanced malnutrition, can be seen.[24] Auscultation of the abdomen may reveal a bruit over the liver, but this finding has low sensitivity, with detection in only 7 out of 240 patients with acute alcoholic hepatitis (AAH) and chronic ALD in one study.[25]

Patients with chronic ALD may be asymptomatic, but more specific symptoms for this condition include those found in patients with cirrhosis or end-stage liver disease, such as confusion (hepatic encephalopathy), abdominal distention or pain (ascites or peritonitis), and hematemesis (variceal bleeding).[26] Physical examination findings in chronic ALD generally are similar to those found in cirrhosis from other causes including spider angiomata, classically found on the face, neck, and upper trunk.[27] The number and size of these lesions is often mediated by the severity of liver disease, which in turn affects levels of estradiol and testosterone; gynecomastia and testicular atrophy from hypogonadism may also be seen. Dupuytren contractures, or palmar fibromatosis of the fourth and fifth fingers, may suggest cirrhosis from alcohol as opposed to other causes, although genetics and occupation may explain this finding in some patients.[28] Palmar erythema is common and is usually most pronounced over the hypothenar and thenar eminences.[27] Parotid enlargement, clubbing of the fingers, peripheral neuropathy, caput medusae, Terry nails (white appearance to proximal two-thirds of nail plate), and Muehrcke lines (horizontal white bands separated by normal color on fingernails) are other findings in chronic ALD.[8]

Overlap of some symptoms and signs, especially between AAH and chronic ALD, may aid the clinician in making not only an accurate diagnosis, but also a general prognosis at the bedside. Jaundice, which has many causes, is more likely to be hepatocellular in origin if there are concurrent findings of chronic ALD, including caput medusae (likelihood ratio [LR], 17.5), palmar erythema (LR, 9.8), spider angiomata (LR, 4.9), ascites (LR, 4.4), or splenomegaly (LR, 2.9).[27] The finding of hepatic encephalopathy in patients with chronic ALD has been associated with higher rates of mortality compared with any other symptom.[29] Other findings that have been associated with an increased 1-year mortality are ascites, spider angiomata, caput medusae, edema, and weakness.[30]

LABORATORY FINDINGS

Concurrent with the physical examination, objective data from laboratory, imaging, and histologic studies are nearly always required to confirm a diagnosis of ALD. Similar to the physical examination, different subsets of ALD (AFLD, AH, and chronic ALD) have some shared and some specific laboratory findings. No one laboratory test confirms or excludes ALD, thus requiring the clinician to understand the relevance and utility of each test for a given patient. The relative sensitivity, specificity, and positive predictive value of selected laboratory tests in the diagnosis of ALD are displayed in **Table 2**.

In AFLD, liver enzymes may range from normal to modestly elevated aspartate aminotransferase (AST) and alanine aminotransferase (ALT). Similar results may be noted in non-AFLD, and a history of prior alcohol use may therefore be the only clue to the diagnosis of AFLD.[31] Furthermore, it must be recognized that AFLD and non-AFLD can occur concomitantly in the same patient, making it challenging in assigning relative contribution from each entity to the clinical presentation.

AH often causes elevations in AST and ALT, but with AST levels usually less than 300 unit/L and rarely greater than 500 unit/L, beyond which other causes of hepatitis are more likely.[24] Typically, the AST/ALT ratio is greater than 2, caused in part by a deficiency of pyridoxal 5'-phosphate, a cofactor of enzymatic activity in the production of ALT.[32] Some have suggested a genetic impact on the AST/ALT ratio, with African American and Hispanic patients with AH more likely to have an AST/ALT ratio greater than 2.[33] Total bilirubin levels in AH generally average around 15 mg/dL, but can be much higher.[24,34] γ-Glutamyltransferase (GGT) levels are also frequently elevated in

Table 2
Sensitivity, specificity, positive predictive value, and negative predictive value of selected laboratory tests in the diagnosis of ALD

Laboratory Test	Relevant ALD Subtypes	Value	Comment
AST, ALT[46,49]	AFLD AAH Chronic ALD	Sn: 35%–50% Sp: 38%–86%	Limited sensitivity More accurate age 30–60
GGT[4,46,47,82–84]	AAH	Sn: 71%–73% Sp: 18%–75% PPV: 82%–92% NPV: 33%–40%	Helpful in early ALD Cheaper than CDT Increased by obesity
MCV[4,46,82,83]	AAH Chronic ALD	Sn: 52%–64% Sp: 66%–85% PPV: 73%–78% NPV: 70%–76%	Elevation may suggest long-standing ALD Insensitive in detecting relapse
CDT[4,46,81]	AAH Chronic ALD	Sn: 69%–88% Sp: 52%–97%	Limited or no use in some laboratories Expensive May help distinguish ALD from non-ALD Many false positive
Mitochondrial AST[48]	Chronic ALD	Sn: 93% NPV: 82%–100%	Limited or no use in some laboratories Good NPV
ETG[45,49]	AAH	Sn: near 100% Sp: near 100%	Present in all body fluids but urine easiest to test Very sensitive, so high false-positive rate because of inadvertent use of alcohol-containing products (ie, mouthwash, hand sanitizers)

Abbreviations: ALT, alanine aminotransferase; AST, aspartate aminotransferase; CDT, carbohydrate-deficient transferrin; ETG, ethyl glucuronide; GGT, γ-glutamyltransferase; MCV, mean red cell volume; NPV, negative predictive value; PPV, positive predictive value; Sn, sensitivity; Sp, specificity.

AH and remain generally more cost-effective than other bioassays.[35] GGT may be especially helpful in identifying early forms of AAH, but is less helpful in chronic ALD because elevations can occur with liver fibrosis of any cause.[36,37]

There are many non-liver-specific laboratory indices that suggest a diagnosis of severe AH. The white blood cell count is generally elevated higher than 20,000 K/µL, but more severe elevations may be seen and are associated with a poor prognosis.[34,38] The mean red cell volume is often elevated, which occurs as a direct effect from long-standing alcoholism causing malnutrition and increased lipid deposition in red blood cells. Ferritin and serum transferrin levels are frequently elevated in AH, which is thought to be in part secondary to suppression of hepcidin synthesis by alcohol.[16] These elevated levels should not prompt a reflexive work-up for hemochromatosis, but further evaluation for hemochromatosis may be considered in the appropriate clinical context.[16] The international normalized ratio may be elevated secondary to a disruption of coagulation factors caused by inflammation or significant hepatic dysfunction. Serum creatinine and serum triglycerides may be elevated, with the former suggesting the need to consider the development of hepatorenal syndrome. Specific nutritional deficiencies (magnesium, phosphorous, vitamin A, vitamin D, thiamine, folate, zinc) may provide further indirect clues to the diagnosis of AAH.

Chronic ALD is often suggested by some of the general biochemical abnormalities found in cirrhosis from other causes, such as coagulopathy; thrombocytopenia, which is often compounded by chronic alcoholism caused by bone marrow suppression; and hypoalbuminemia. There is some evidence that total bilirubin increases and GGT decreases as severity of ALD increases.[39] An elevated GGT does not exclude chronic ALD, but rather may suggest AH in addition to chronic ALD.[36]

Interest in noninvasive means to assess for fibrosis or chronic ALD has resulted in various specialized applications of laboratory markers. The AST/platelet index, which remains somewhat reliable in predicting fibrosis in patients with hepatitis C, has poor sensitivity for diagnosing fibrosis in patients with chronic ALD.[40,41] The FibroTest, which uses α_2-macroglobulin, haptoglobin, GGT, apolipoprotein A-I, and total bilirubin (corrected for age and sex), seems useful in evaluating for advanced fibrosis in ALD, and is generally comparable with Fibrometer (ARUP laboratories, Salt Lake City, UT) and Hepascore tests.[36,42] Although helpful, a simpler approach to these complex scoring systems includes the more traditional and accessible assessment of platelet count and international normalized ratio. A recent analysis found that a presobriety platelet count of less than 70 cells/mm^3 has a positive LR of 6.8 in ruling in cirrhosis, whereas a presobriety platelet count of greater than 200 cells/mm^3 has a negative LR of 0.18 in ruling out cirrhosis.[43]

The differential diagnosis of ALD is broad and includes, but is not limited to, acute and chronic viral hepatitis; hemochromatosis; drug-induced injury; ischemic hepatitis; Budd-Chiari syndrome; autoimmune hepatitis; Wilson disease; α_1-antitrypsin deficiency; pregnancy-related injury; and infectious causes, such as pyogenic hepatic abscess.[24] These entities should at least be considered in patients suspected of having ALD because some exist concurrently with ALD, and may affect outcomes and management. For example, hepatitis C and alcohol hasten the progression of liver disease and hepatocellular carcinoma synergistically, and thus hepatitis C should always be tested for in patients with ALD.[44]

NOVEL BIOMARKERS

A positive serum ethanol level confirms acute alcohol use, but because this assay remains positive generally only on the order of hours after ingestion, it is of limited use in most patients with chronic ALD.[45] Therefore, there is a need for more specific biomarkers of AH and chronic ALD. But as with standard biochemical tests, none replace the value of a careful history and examination. Furthermore, many of these biomarkers have not been adopted widely because of their cost and limitations and uncertainty in their performance characteristics.[45–48]

The best-studied of these tests, carbohydrate-deficient transferrin (CDT), correlates with alcohol use, and is based on the fact that chronic alcohol use reduces the number of carbohydrate moieties attached to transferrin.[45,46] CDT can therefore help distinguish ALD from non-ALD, but expense, false-positive rates, and variability of results based on age, weight, and gender limit it from wider use (see **Table 2**).[46,47,49] CDT is also affected by baseline serum transferrin levels, hypertension, and the presence of chronic viral hepatitis or decompensated liver disease.[50] CDT is also not sensitive for modest alcohol use, with data indicating a minimum threshold for detection of 60 g of alcohol daily for weeks.[45]

Ethyl glucuronide (ETG) is a nonoxidative ethanol metabolite that, unlike CDT, is sensitive for even light alcohol use (positive results may be seen with one alcoholic drink consumed), with positive results lasting up to 2 days.[49,51,52] This sensitivity also means higher rates of false-positive results, but ETG remains a promising adjunct in the arsenal of laboratory testing for ALD pending further testing (see **Table 2**).[45,49]

Another newer biomarker, phosphatidyl ethanol, has excellent sensitivity for light to moderate alcohol use and unlike ETG can persist for up to 3 weeks, but more research has been recommended before implementation in clinical settings.[45] Mitochondrial AST, first presented as an option in the evaluation of chronic ALD in the 1980s and useful because of its longer half-life compared with cytosolic AST, has not been widely adopted in clinical practice because of its limited specificity.[48,53]

IMAGING STUDIES

The diagnosis of ALD may also be supported by imaging studies. However, hepatic imaging may only help identify the general presence and degree of liver disease, and does not prove or disprove alcohol as the etiologic mechanism. Imaging modalities are more frequently helpful in excluding other confounding or concurrent diagnoses, such as Budd-Chiari syndrome, portal vein thrombosis, malignancy, or liver abscess.

AFLD may be supported by the findings of steatosis, which are identified on ultrasound, computed tomography (CT), or MRI. A recent meta-analysis including patients with AFLD showed that ultrasound had 85% sensitivity, 94% specificity, positive LR of 13, and negative LR of 0.16 for steatosis.[54] MRI had the highest specificity (up to 97.4%) and similar sensitivity compared with other imaging modalities.[55–57] However, despite having lower specificity than MRI, ultrasound is generally cheaper and more widely available, and as such remains more broadly used as the preferred screening tool for steatosis in patients suspected of having early ALD.[58] The application of newer imaging modalities in AFLD remains uncertain. Transient elastography has been used in patients with non-AFLD. It is currently not recommended for the evaluation of AFLD at this point pending further studies.[59]

AH similarly can be evaluated by ultrasound, CT, or MRI. Although there are limited data on the pathognomonic imaging findings in AH, one potential such finding is the "pseudoparallel channel sign," which describes a dilated hepatic artery and a dilated portal venous branch seen by ultrasound with Doppler flowmetry.[60] This finding was observed in 90% of 77 patients with AH, but only 23% of 119 patients with other forms of ALD, and was not detected in 15 patients with non-ALD.[60] Studies measuring the diameter of the hepatic artery (based on the notion that AH results in increased hepatic artery diameter and flow) have shown increases in hepatic artery diameter and peak systolic velocity with AH compared with chronic ALD or non-ALD.[61,62] These findings were shown to correlate reasonably well with Maddrey discriminant function, revealing their potential use as tools in the prognosis of AH.[62] Although these findings are intriguing, there is still no imaging finding that in isolation is sufficient in the diagnosis of AH, and further studies are needed to investigate the use of performing these studies routinely for the diagnosis of AH.

Chronic ALD can be suggested by findings of advanced fibrosis or cirrhosis on ultrasound, CT, MRI, or transient elastography. Most radiographic features of chronic ALD are consistent with those seen in cirrhosis in general, and include hypertrophy of the left lateral segment, attenuation of hepatic vasculature, ascites, splenomegaly, and presence of venous collaterals. There is some evidence that a large caudate lobe, small regenerative nodules, and more frequent visualization of the right posterior hepatic notch are more commonly seen in alcoholic cirrhosis compared with cirrhosis from viral hepatitis, but further studies are needed to confirm these findings.[63] Transient elastography has proven reliability for assessing fibrosis in hepatitis C virus and non-AFLD and may ultimately preclude the need for liver biopsy.[64] However, transient elastography has limitations; in particular, it may be less reliable in patients with active hepatic inflammation, including AH.[65,66] Other imaging techniques that largely remain experimental at this point with limited clinical applicability include MR spectroscopy, technetium sulfur colloid liver-spleen scan, and perfused hepatic mass imaging.

LIVER BIOPSY

Histologic assessment via liver biopsy in ALD is no longer routinely obtained, especially given the excellent pretest probability of making an accurate diagnosis of ALD based on clinical assessment alone.[67] However, liver biopsy should still be considered in select scenarios:

- Uncertainty about the diagnosis of ALD, either via an incomplete or inconsistent history, or equivocal laboratory or imaging findings
- Concern about a coexisting liver injury, which may occur in 20% of patients with ALD[2,68]
- To confirm a diagnosis or assess the severity of ALD before starting treatment, particularly corticosteroids[2,7,69]
- To assess for chronicity, or fibrosis, and thereby provide a more accurate prognosis for the patient (although transient elastography may supplant biopsy for this indication in the future)
- Enrollment in a clinical trial requires liver biopsy to enhance patient homogenization[7,70]

Others arguments in favor of liver biopsy include assessing for evidence of active AH (implying recent alcohol use) before liver transplant, and to obtain histologic evidence of ALD to convince patients to quit drinking alcohol, but these indications have not been widely adopted.[16,19]

When liver biopsy is pursued, either transvenous or percutaneous approaches are possible, with clinician preference and resource availability often dictating the approach. A transvenous route is generally recommended if the patient has ascites or significant coagulopathy to reduce risk of complications (ie, bleeding), although the magnitude of reduction of these complications remains uncertain.[71]

The findings of liver biopsy in ALD include microvesicular or macrovesicular steatosis, megamitochondria, an increased number of autophagic vacuoles, Mallory-Denk bodies, portal inflammation, and proliferation of smooth endoplasmic reticulum.[9,72] Ongoing alcohol use by patients who have histologic findings of ALD is associated with progression to fibrosis in 20%, further reinforcing the importance of alcohol cessation.[73] For more information on the findings of liver biopsy in ALD, please see Alpert L, Hart J: The Pathology of Alcoholic Liver Disease, in this issue.

Histologic findings in AH are fairly well characterized and generally include four main findings (**Fig. 1**). The first and most common finding is macrovesicular steatosis with or without microsteatosis, which generally connotes early liver injury and is also found in AFLD and nonalcoholic steatohepatitis.[74] Historically, steatosis was thought to represent a benign feature of ALD, but is currently believed to predispose to the development of chronic ALD.[73] The second is a neutrophilic predominant inflammatory pattern, which is more common in alcoholic than in viral hepatitis.[2,7] The third is fibrosis and associated lobular distortion, which often starts in the perivenular regions in early stages of the disease.[2,75] The fourth is hepatocellular ballooning (European Association for the Study of Liver). Patients may have one, some, or all of these findings, and 14% of patients with AH may have none of these findings.[7,74]

Another common finding in 75% of patients with AH is the presence of Mallory-Denk bodies (formerly called Mallory hyaline), which are eosinophilic collections of

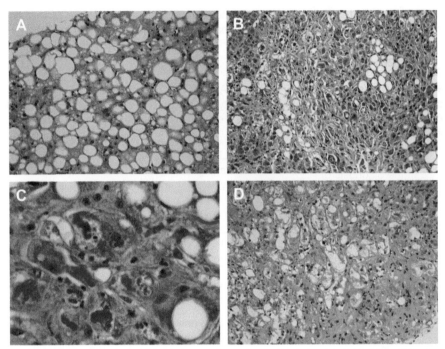

Fig. 1. Histologic findings in AAH. (*A*) Macrovesicular steatosis (H&E, original magnification ×200). (*B*) Fibrosis and associated lobular distortion (Trichrome, original magnification ×200). (*C*) Mallory-Denk bodies (H&E, original magnification ×600). (*D*) Hepatocellular ballooning (H&E, original magnification ×200). (*Courtesy of* Christian Lanciault, MD, PhD, Oregon Health and Science University.)

intracellular structural protein debris.[72] These may suggest active alcohol use, but because they can also be seen in nonalcoholic steatohepatitis, their specificity remains limited.[7,76] Other histologic features of AH include bile duct proliferation and cholestasis.

Diagnosis of AH often requires an assessment of prognosis, for which many scoring systems exist. A histologic scoring system was recently devised and suggests that degree of fibrosis, type of neutrophil infiltration, type of bilirubinostasis, and presence of megamitochondria were independently associated with 90-day mortality.[77] Interestingly, lobular fibrosis, hepatocellular ballooning, the presence of Mallory-Denk bodies, and the degree of steatosis were not significantly associated with mortality. Indications for and clinical relevance of these and other nonhistologic scoring systems should be individualized, but are frequently helpful in the management and counseling of patients with AH.

Micronodular cirrhosis is the most common end-stage finding in chronic ALD, but macronodular cirrhosis and mixed micronodular/macronodular cirrhosis may be seen.[78] A past history of alcoholic steatohepatitis remains the most important risk factor for the development of histologic findings in chronic ALD.[79,80]

SUMMARY

ALD remains an increasingly important clinical entity, with an increasing prevalence and growing economic burden. The approach to the diagnosis of ALD requires an accurate patient history and detailed physical examination. An effective patient history includes a detailed scrutiny of the quantity and pattern of alcohol use and the medical, social, and economic consequences of this use. Nonetheless, it is equally important to obtain this history in a nonjudgmental, empathetic way to establish an effective patient-provider relationship to maximize diagnostic accuracy and therapeutic effectiveness. The physical examination remains an important tool in helping to clarify the subtypes of ALD present. Clinicians should also maintain an understanding of the value, relevance, and applicability of routine laboratory indices, imaging studies, and histopathology. Novel biomarkers, scoring systems, and imaging modalities are improving the ability to diagnose and manage ALD, but for most practicing clinicians, these remain novel, and not routinely implemented. Liver biopsy has become sparingly used in the diagnosis of ALD, but retains its critical importance in specific scenarios and as the established gold standard in the diagnosis of ALD.

REFERENCES

1. Lefkowitch JH. Morphology of alcoholic liver disease. Clin Liver Dis 2005;9(1): 37–53.
2. O'Shea RS, Dasarathy S, McCullough AJ, et al. Alcoholic liver disease. Hepatology 2010;51:307.
3. Jinjuvadia R, Liangpunsakul S, Translational Research and Evolving Alcoholic Hepatitis Treatment Consortium. Trends in alcoholic hepatitis-related hospitalizations, financial burden, and mortality in the United States. J Clin Gastroenterol 2014;49(6):506–11.
4. Saitz R. Clinical practice. Unhealthy alcohol use. N Engl J Med 2005;352(6):596.
5. Cohen SM, Ahn J. Review article: the diagnosis and management of alcoholic hepatitis. Aliment Pharmacol Ther 2009;30:3.
6. Chalasani N, Younossi Z, Lavine JE, et al. The diagnosis and management of non-alcoholic fatty liver disease: Practice guideline by the American Association for the Study of Liver Diseases, American College of Gastroenterology, and the American Gastroenterological Association. Am J Gastroenterol 2012;107(6): 811–26.
7. European Association for the Study of Liver. EASL clinical practical guidelines: management of alcoholic liver disease. J Hepatol 2012;57:399.
8. McCullough AJ, O'Connor JF. Alcoholic liver disease: proposed recommendations for the American College of Gastroenterology. Am J Gastroenterol 1998; 93(11):2022–36.
9. Rubin E, Lieber CS. Alcohol-induced hepatic injury in nonalcoholic volunteers. N Engl J Med 1968;278(16):869–76.
10. Bellentani S, Saccoccio G, Costa G, et al. Drinking habits as cofactors of risk for alcohol induced liver damage. The Dionysos Study Group. Gut 1997;41:845.
11. Stinson FS, Grant BF, Dufour MC. The critical dimension of ethnicity in liver cirrhosis mortality statistics. Alcohol Clin Exp Res 2001;25:1181–7.
12. Chedid A, Mendenhall CL, Gartside P, et al. Prognostic factors in alcoholic liver disease. VA Cooperative Study Group. Am J Gastroenterol 1991;86:210.
13. Levine J. The relative value of consultation, questionnaires and laboratory investigation in the identification of excessive alcohol consumption. Alcohol Alcohol 1990;25:539–53.
14. U.S. Preventive Services Task Force (USPSTF). Screening and behavioral counselling interventions in primary care to reduce alcohol misuse. Recommendation

Statement. 2004. Available at: http://www.uspreventiveservicestaskforce.org. Accessed May 17, 2015.

15. Livingston M, Callinan S. Underreporting in alcohol surveys: whose drinking is underestimated? J Stud Alcohol Drugs 2015;76(1):158–64.

16. Choi G, Runyon BA. Alcoholic hepatitis: a clinician's guide. Clin Liver Dis 2012; 16:371.

17. Gleeson D, Jones JS, McFarlane E, et al. Severity of alcohol dependence in decompensated alcoholic liver disease: comparison with heavy drinkers without liver disease and relationship to family drinking history. Alcohol Alcohol 2009; 44(4):392–7.

18. Jauhar S, Talwalkar JA, Schneekloth T, et al. Analysis of factors that predict alcohol relapse following liver transplantation. Liver Transpl 2004;10(3):408–11.

19. Levitsky J, Mailliard ME. Diagnosis and therapy of alcoholic liver disease. Semin Liver Dis 2004;24(3):233–47.

20. Zoli M, Magalotti D, Grimaldi M, et al. Physical examination of the liver: is it still worth it? Am J Gastroenterol 1995;90:1428–32.

21. Espinosa P, Ducot B, Pelletier G, et al. Interobserver agreement in the physical diagnosis of alcoholic liver disease. Dig Dis Sci 1987;32:244–7.

22. Baraona E, Leo MA, Borowsky SA, et al. Alcoholic hepatomegaly: accumulation of protein in the liver. Science 1975;190:794.

23. Lischner MW, Alexander JF, Galambos JT. Natural history of alcoholic hepatitis. I. The acute disease. Am J Dig Dis 1971;16(6):481–94.

24. Lucey MR, Mathurin P, Morgan TR. Alcoholic hepatitis. N Engl J Med 2009; 360(26):2758–69.

25. Zoneraich S, Zoneraich O. Diagnostic significance of abdominal arterial murmurs in liver and pancreatic disease. A phonoarteriographic study. Angiology 1971;22: 197–205.

26. Tandon P, Garcia-Tsao G. Bacterial infections, sepsis, and multiorgan failure in cirrhosis. Semin Liver Dis 2008;28:26–42.

27. McGee S. Evidence-based physical diagnosis. Philadelphia: Saunder-Elsevier; 2007.

28. Burge P, Hoy G, Regan P, et al. Smoking, alcohol and the risk of Dupuytren's contracture. J Bone Joint Surg Br 1997;79(2):206.

29. Jepsen P, Ott P, Andersen PK, et al. Clinical course of alcoholic liver cirrhosis: a Danish population-based cohort study. Hepatology 2010;51(5):1675–82.

30. Orrego H, Israel Y, Blake JE, et al. Assessment of prognostic factors in alcoholic liver disease: toward a global quantitative expression of severity. Hepatology 1983;3:896–905.

31. Sorbi D, Boynton J, Lindor KD. The ratio of aspartate aminotransferase to alanine aminotransferase: potential value in differentiating nonalcoholic steatohepatitis from alcoholic liver disease. Am J Gastroenterol 1999;94(4):1018–22.

32. Diehl AM, Potter J, Boitnott J, et al. Relationship between pyridoxal 5'-phosphate deficiency and aminotransferase levels in alcoholic hepatitis. Gastroenterology 1984;86(4):632.

33. Stewart SH. Racial and ethnic differences in alcohol associated aspartate aminotransferase and gamma-glutamyltransferase elevation. Arch Intern Med 2002; 162:2236–9.

34. Nguyen-Khac E, Thevenot T, Piquet MA, et al. Glucocorticoids plus N-acetylcysteine in severe alcoholic hepatitis. N Engl J Med 2011;365:1781.

35. Seitz HK. Additive effects of moderate drinking and obesity on serum gamma-glutamyl transferase. Am J Clin Nutr 2006;83:1252–3.

36. Imbert-Bismut F, Ratziu V, Pieroni L, et al. Biochemical markers of liver fibrosis in patients with hepatitis C virus infection: a prospective study. Lancet 2001;357: 1069–75.
37. Menon K, Gores G, Shah V. Pathogenesis, diagnosis, and treatment of alcoholic liver disease. Mayo Clin Proc 2001;76:1021–9.
38. Mitchell RG, Michael M 3rd, Sandidge D. High mortality among patients with the leukemoid reaction and alcoholic hepatitis. South Med J 1991;84:281.
39. Poynard T, Zourabichvili O, Hilpert G, et al. Prognostic value of total serum bilirubin/gamma-glutamyl transpeptidase ratio in cirrhotic patients. Hepatology 1984;4(2):324–7.
40. Lieber CS, Weiss DG, Morgan TR, et al. Aspartate aminotransferase to platelet ratio index in patients with alcoholic liver fibrosis. Am J Gastroenterol 2006;101: 1500–8.
41. Toniutto P, Fabris C, Bitetto D, et al. Role of AST to platelet ratio index in the detection of liver fibrosis in patients with recurrent hepatitis C after liver transplantation. J Gastroenterol Hepatol 2007;22(11):1904–8.
42. Naveau S, Gaude G, Asnacios A, et al. Diagnostic and prognostic values of noninvasive biomarkers of fibrosis in patients with alcoholic liver disease. Hepatology 2009;49:97–105.
43. Murali AR, Attar BM, Katz A, et al. Utility of platelet count for predicting cirrhosis in alcoholic liver disease: model for identifying cirrhosis in a US Population. J Gen Intern Med 2015;30(8):1112–7.
44. Safdar K, Schiff ER. Alcohol and hepatitis C. Semin Liver Dis 2004;24(3):305–15.
45. Center for Substance Abuse Treatment. The role of biomarkers in the treatment of alcohol use disorders, 2012 revision, vol. 11. Rockville, MD: Substance Abuse and Mental Health Services Administration Advisory; Spring; 2012. 2.
46. Bell H, Tallaksen CM, Try K, et al. Carbohydrate-deficient transferrin and other markers of high alcohol consumption: a study of 502 patients admitted consecutively to a medical department. Alcohol Clin Exp Res 1994;18:1103–8.
47. Hock B, Schwarz M, Domke I, et al. Validity of carbohydrate-deficient transferrin (%CDT), gamma-glutamyltransferase (gamma-GT) and mean corpuscular erythrocyte volume (MCV) as biomarkers for chronic alcohol abuse: a study in patients with alcohol dependence and liver disorders of non-alcoholic and alcoholic origin. Addiction 2005;100(10):1477–86.
48. Nalpas B, Vassault A, Le Guillou A, et al. Serum activity of mitochondrial aspartate aminotransferase: a sensitive marker of alcoholism with or without alcoholic hepatitis. Hepatology 1984;4(5):893–6.
49. Litten R, Bradley AM, Moss HB, et al. Alcohol biomarkers in applied settings: recent advances and future research opportunities. Alcohol Clin Exp Res 2010; 34(6):955–67.
50. DiMartini A, Day N, Lane T, et al. Carbohydrate deficient transferrin in abstaining patients with end-stage liver disease. Alcohol Clin Exp Res 2001;25:1729–33.
51. Kissack JC, Bishop J, Roper AL. Ethylglucuronide as a biomarker for ethanol detection. Pharmacotherapy 2008;28(6):769–81.
52. Cabarcos P, Álvarez I, Tabernero MJ, et al. Determination of direct alcohol markers: a review. Anal Bioanal Chem 2015;407(17):4907–25.
53. Dufour DR, Lott JA, Nolte FS, et al. Diagnosis and monitoring of hepatic injury. I. Performance characteristics of laboratory tests. Clin Chem 2000;46(12):2027–49.
54. Hernaez R, Lazo M, Bonekamp S, et al. Diagnostic accuracy and reliability of ultrasonography for the detection of fatty liver: a meta-analysis. Hepatology 2011; 54(3):1082–90.

55. Bohte AE, van Werven JR, Bipat S, et al. The diagnostic accuracy of US, CT, MRI and 1H-MRS for the evaluation of hepatic steatosis compared with liver biopsy: a meta-analysis. Eur Radiol 2011;21(1):87–97.

56. d'Assignies G, Ruel M, Khiat A, et al. Noninvasive quantitation of human liver steatosis using magnetic resonance and bioassay methods. Eur Radiol 2009; 19(8):2033–40.

57. Zhong L, Chen JJ, Chen J, et al. Nonalcoholic fatty liver disease: quantitative assessment of liver fat content by computed tomography, magnetic resonance imaging and proton magnetic resonance spectroscopy. J Dig Dis 2009;10(4): 315–20.

58. Ratziu V, Bellentani S, Cortez-Pinto H, et al. A position statement on NAFLD/NASH based on the EASL 2009 special conference. J Hepatol 2010;53:372–84.

59. Cocciolillo S, Parruti G, Marzio L. CEUS and Fibroscan in non-alcoholic fatty liver disease and non-alcoholic steatohepatitis. World J Hepatol 2014;6(7):496–503.

60. Sumino Y, Kravetz D, Kanel GC, et al. Ultrasonographic diagnosis of acute alcoholic hepatitis 'pseudoparallel channel sign' of intrahepatic artery dilatation. Gastroenterology 1993;105:1477.

61. Han SH, Rice S, Cohen SM, et al. Duplex Doppler ultrasound of the hepatic artery in patients with acute alcoholic hepatitis. J Clin Gastroenterol 2002;34(5):573–7.

62. Abhilash H, Mukunda M, Sunil P, et al. Hepatic artery duplex Doppler ultrasound in severe alcoholic hepatitis and correlation with Maddrey's discriminant function. Ann Gastroenterol 2015;28(2):271–5.

63. Okazaki H, Ito K, Fujita T, et al. Discrimination of alcoholic from virus-induced cirrhosis on MR imaging. AJR Am J Roentgenol 2000;175(6):1677–81.

64. Janssens F, de Suray N, Piessevaux H, et al. Can transient elastography replace liver histology for determination of advanced fibrosis in alcoholic patients: a real-life study. J Clin Gastroenterol 2010;44:575–82.

65. Trabut JB, Thépot V, Nalpas B, et al. Rapid decline of liver stiffness following alcohol withdrawal in heavy drinkers. Alcohol Clin Exp Res 2012;36:1407.

66. Mueller S, Millonig G, Sarovska L, et al. Increased liver stiffness in alcoholic liver disease: differentiating fibrosis from steatohepatitis. World J Gastroenterol 2010; 16(8):966–72.

67. Van Ness MM, Diehl AM. Is liver biopsy useful in the evaluation of patients with chronically elevated liver enzymes? Ann Intern Med 1989;111:473.

68. Levin DM, Baker AL, Riddell RH, et al. Nonalcoholic liver disease. Overlooked causes of liver injury in patients with heavy alcohol consumption. Am J Med 1979;66(3):429–34.

69. Poynard T, Ratziu V, Bedossa P. Appropriateness of liver biopsy. Can J Gastroenterol 2000;14:543–8.

70. Dhanda AD, Collins PL, McCune AC. Is liver biopsy necessary in the management of alcoholic hepatitis? World J Gastroenterol 2013;19(44):7825–9.

71. Grant A, Neuberger J. Guidelines on the use of liver biopsy in clinical practice. British Society of Gastroenterology. Gut 1999;45(Suppl 4):IV1–11.

72. French SW, Nash J, Shitabata P, et al. Pathology of alcoholic liver disease. VA Cooperative Study Group 119. Semin Liver Dis 1993;13:154–69.

73. Teli MR, Day CP, Burt AD, et al. Determinants of progression to cirrhosis or fibrosis in pure alcoholic fatty liver. Lancet 1995;346:987–90.

74. Naveau S, Giraud V, Borotto E, et al. Excess weight risk factor for alcoholic liver disease. Hepatology 1997;25:108–11.

75. Savolainen V, Perola M, Lalu K, et al. Early perivenular fibrogenesis–precirrhotic lesions among moderate alcohol consumers and chronic alcoholics. J Hepatol 1995;23:524–31.
76. Bacon BR, Farahvash MJ, Janney CG, et al. Nonalcoholic steatohepatitis: an expanded clinical entity. Gastroenterology 1994;107:1103.
77. Altamirano J, Miquel R, Katoonizadeh A, et al. A histologic scoring system for prognosis of patients with alcoholic hepatitis. Gastroenterology 2014;146:1231.
78. Hall PD. Pathological spectrum of alcoholic liver disease. Alcohol Alcohol 1994;2: 303–13.
79. Mathurin P, Beuzin F, Louvet A, et al. Fibrosis progression occurs in a subgroup of heavy drinkers with typical histological features. Aliment Pharmacol Ther 2007; 25:1047–54.
80. Parés A, Caballería J, Bruguera M, et al. Histological course of alcoholic hepatitis. Influence of abstinence, sex and extent of hepatic damage. J Hepatol 1986;2:33.
81. Stibler H. Carbohydrate-deficient transferrin in serum: a new marker of potentially harmful alcohol consumption reviewed. Clin Chem 1991;37(12):2029–37.
82. Pasqualetti P, Festuccia V, MacCarone C, et al. Diagnostic value of gamma glutamyl transpeptidase and the mean corpuscular volume in chronic hepatitis of alcoholic etiology. Minerva Med 1995;86(10):395–402 [in Italian].
83. Pol S, Poynard T, Bedossa P, et al. Diagnostic value of serum gamma-glutamyl-transferase activity and mean corpuscular volume in alcoholic patients with or without cirrhosis. Alcohol Clin Exp Res 1990;14(2):250–4.
84. Alatalo P, Koivisto H, Puukka K, et al. Biomarkers of liver status in heavy drinkers, moderate drinkers and abstainers. Alcohol Alcohol 2009;44(2):199–203.

The Pathology of Alcoholic Liver Disease

Lindsay Alpert, MD*, John Hart, MD

KEYWORDS

- Steatosis • Alcoholic steatohepatitis • Ballooning degeneration • Cholestasis
- Sinusoidal fibrosis • Cirrhosis

KEY POINTS

- Macrovesicular steatosis is a common pathologic feature present in a wide variety of inflammatory, toxic, congenital, metabolic, and neoplastic diseases that affect the liver, including alcoholic liver disease.
- There is a continuum between macrovesicular steatosis and steatohepatitis, but when evidence of parenchymal inflammation and hepatocyte injury is present, a diagnosis of steatohepatitis is appropriate.
- Histologic distinction between alcoholic and nonalcoholic fatty liver disease is often impossible, but certain morphologic features are highly suggestive of alcohol as the source of liver injury.
- Accurate staging of fibrosis in cases of alcoholic liver disease is important for clinical management and prognostic purposes.
- Many patients with alcoholic liver disease have additional sources of liver injury, and detection of coexisting conditions has important therapeutic implications.

INTRODUCTION

In his seminal treatise *On Diseases of the Liver* from 1857, British physician George Budd vividly describes[1]

> ...a liver...taken from a drunkard...in a state of cirrhosis, as well as of fatty degeneration, [that] in consequence presented [with] a very remarkable "hob-nailed" appearance, from the nodules of cirrhosis being enlarged by the accumulation of oil. A portion of it blazed when thrown into the fire, and a particle from the lobular substance had under the microscope almost the appearance of ordinary fat tissue, from the number and size of the oil-globules it contained.

Although evaluation of liver flammability is no longer a routine element of the diagnostic work-up for alcoholic liver disease, the gross and microscopic features of this

Disclosure Statement: The authors have nothing to disclose.
Department of Pathology, The University of Chicago, 5841 South Maryland Avenue, MC 6101, Chicago, IL 60637, USA
* Corresponding author.
E-mail address: Lindsay.Alpert@uchospitals.edu

Clin Liver Dis 20 (2016) 473–489
http://dx.doi.org/10.1016/j.cld.2016.02.006
liver.theclinics.com

condition remain striking to this day. Alcoholic liver disease is still one of the leading causes of liver failure in the United States and worldwide, and given the potentially reversible nature of this condition, the pathology of alcoholic liver disease remains a topic worthy of review.

The term "alcoholic liver disease" encompasses a spectrum of pathologic conditions ranging from isolated steatosis to established cirrhosis. Within this spectrum, varying degrees of inflammation, hepatocyte ballooning and necrosis, cholestasis, and fibrosis may be encountered. This article reviews the characteristic histologic features of the many forms of alcoholic liver disease.

STEATOSIS (FATTY LIVER)

Macrovesicular steatosis (**Fig. 1**) is a common pathologic feature present in a wide variety of inflammatory, toxic, congenital, metabolic, and neoplastic diseases that affect the liver. Although other causes of clear cytoplasmic vacuolization of hepatocytes must always be kept in mind, most do not cause displacement of the nucleus to the cell membrane, which is the characteristic feature of macrovesicular steatosis. A component of microvesicular steatosis, or small droplets of fat that do not cause nuclear displacement, may also be present (**Fig. 2**), particularly in the setting of binge drinking with acute decompensation (see later discussion of alcoholic foamy degeneration). The pathogenesis of lipid deposition in hepatocytes is beyond the scope of this discussion.

Steatosis in alcoholic liver disease is usually present in a centrilobular distribution (**Fig. 3**), although it may also be diffuse. Abstinence from ethanol is said to lead to disappearance of steatosis, although the duration of abstinence required for complete resolution of steatosis is hard to pinpoint. Certainly most patients with alcoholic cirrhosis who abstain to be listed for liver transplantation have minimal or no steatosis evident at 6 to 12 months after cessation of alcohol use, when the native liver is removed. In patients with only alcoholic steatosis, disappearance of lipid usually occurs within 1 to 3 months. However, small lipogranulomas, or aggregates of histiocytes and inflammatory cells surrounding extracellular lipid droplets, may be seen in the lobules or portal tracts long after the steatosis resolves. These

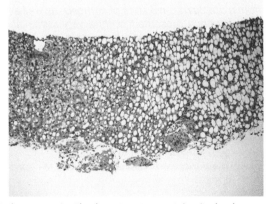

Fig. 1. Macrovesicular steatosis. The hepatocytes contain single clear vacuoles that occupy almost all the cytoplasm. There is no lobular inflammation, hepatocyte ballooning degeneration or necrosis, or Mallory-Denk bodies, ruling out steatohepatitis (hematoxylin-eosin, original magnification ×40).

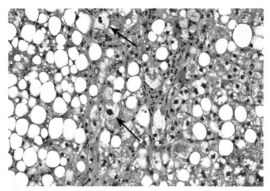

Fig. 2. Macrovesicular versus microvesicular steatosis. The hepatocyte nuclei are displaced to the periphery of the cell by the single large lipid vacuoles in macrovesicular fat. The nucleus remains centralized with microvesicular steatosis (*arrows*) (hematoxylin-eosin, original magnification ×100).

lipogranulomas apparently form as a result of release of lipid from ruptured steatotic hepatocytes.[2] A similar process can also give rise to foamy histiocytes within portal tracts, which may be the only remaining sign of prior steatosis in some cases.

ALCOHOLIC STEATOHEPATITIS (ALCOHOLIC HEPATITIS)

Certain histologic features, when present in addition to steatosis, create a characteristic pattern that is referred to as steatohepatitis. These features were first recognized in patients with alcoholic liver disease,[3] although identical histologic features can be seen in patients without any history of alcohol ingestion, in which case the term nonalcoholic steatohepatitis (NASH) is used.[4] The major features of steatohepatitis are hepatocyte ballooning degeneration, lobular inflammation (especially neutrophils), Mallory-Denk bodies, individual hepatocyte necrosis/dropout, and glycogenated hepatocyte nuclei.[5] Mild portal mononuclear cell infiltrates may also be present.

Hepatocyte ballooning degeneration and acidophil bodies are the primary histologic features of hepatocyte injury in alcoholic steatohepatitis. Hepatocyte ballooning, which occurs primarily in the perivenular areas, can be difficult to recognize in the face of significant macrovesicular steatosis. The retention of a centrally placed nucleus is the best clue to recognizing a ballooned hepatocyte. In addition, although these cells exhibit clear vacuolization, strands or clumps of cytoplasm are usually also evident, often in a spider web pattern (**Fig. 4**). Acidophil bodies (also known as Councilman bodies) are apoptotic hepatocytes that are recognized by their shrunken size,

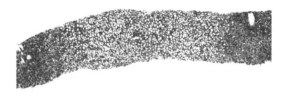

Fig. 3. Centrilobular steatosis. A distinct centrilobular distribution of the steatosis is evident, with sparing of the periportal regions at each end of the biopsy (hematoxylin-eosin, original magnification ×20).

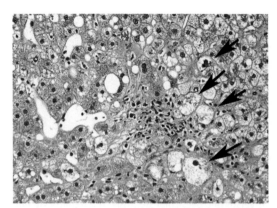

Fig. 4. Ballooned hepatocytes. The cells are enlarged and the cytoplasm is wispy, with centrally placed nuclei (*arrows*) (hematoxylin-eosin, original magnification ×100).

dense eosinophilic cytoplasm, and pyknotic nucleus (**Fig. 5**). Like macrovesicular steatosis, ballooned hepatocytes and acidophils bodies are not specific to alcoholic liver disease, but instead are seen in a range of inflammatory, toxic, and metabolic conditions.

Mallory-Denk bodies (alcoholic hyaline), when present, are almost always seen within ballooned hepatocytes (**Fig. 6**).[5,6] These bodies represent condensation of denatured cytokeratin filaments, and are associated with the chaperone molecule ubiquitin. Immunohistochemical stains using CK7, CK18, CK19, p62, or ubiquitin antibodies highlight the presence of Mallory-Denk bodies (**Fig. 7**), but these stains are not necessary in routine diagnostic practice.[7] Mallory-Denk bodies are not pathognomonic for alcoholic hepatitis. They are often present in the periportal zone in chronic cholestatic conditions and Wilson disease, and in the centrilobular zones in NASH and amiodarone toxicity.

Lobular neutrophilic infiltrates are also characteristic of alcoholic steatohepatitis. Neutrophils can sometimes be seen surrounding acidophil bodies and hepatocytes containing prominent Mallory-Denk bodies (**Fig. 8**). Scattered small clusters of mononuclear cells are also often present, and they may mark foci of individual hepatocyte dropout, which can be highlighted using a reticulin stain.

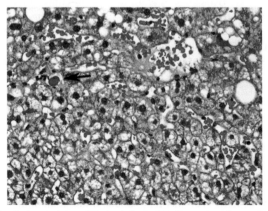

Fig. 5. Acidophil body (*arrow*) in mild steatohepatitis (hematoxylin-eosin, original magnification ×200).

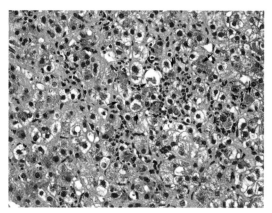

Fig. 6. Mallory-Denk bodies. Many of the ballooned hepatocytes in this field contain Mallory-Denk bodies (*arrows*) (hematoxylin-eosin, original magnification ×100).

Mild portal mononuclear cell infiltrates are a common feature in older series of cases of alcoholic steatohepatitis reported in the literature, but these studies were performed before the availability of tests for infection with hepatitis C virus. Nevertheless, it is clear that portal inflammation of some degree is present in many cases where chronic viral hepatitis has been excluded.[8] The presence of dense portal infiltrates, however, should lead the pathologist to raise the possibility of superimposed chronic hepatitis.

Distinction Between Steatosis and Steatohepatitis

There is a fluid continuum between macrovesicular steatosis and steatohepatitis, and the precise moment of transition from one condition to the next is likely indiscernible. When there is evidence of parenchymal inflammation and hepatocyte injury in addition to steatosis, a diagnosis of alcoholic steatohepatitis can be rendered. However, there are currently no generally recognized criteria that sharply delineate the combination and/or severity of changes necessary to make the diagnosis of steatohepatitis, as opposed to simple macrovesicular steatosis. In some early reports, a combination of macrovesicular steatosis and spotty lobular inflammation was enough to classify

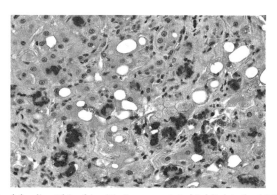

Fig. 7. Mallory-Denk bodies. This ubiquitin immunostain highlights the Mallory-Denk bodies (ubiquitin, original magnification ×200).

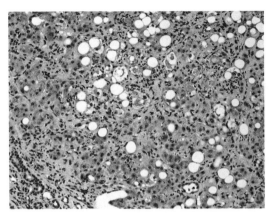

Fig. 8. Lobular neutrophilic infiltrates. The neutrophils typically surround the hepatocytes containing the Mallory-Denk bodies. This degree of neutrophilic inflammation is beyond that expected in nonalcoholic steatohepatitis (hematoxylin-eosin, original magnification ×100).

a case as steatohepatitis. More recently, additional evidence of hepatocyte injury has been required, including hepatocyte ballooning, Mallory-Denk body formation, or sinusoidal fibrosis. However, none of these studies clearly quantify the minimal severity of these changes necessary to make the diagnosis of steatohepatitis. Some have argued that requiring the presence of fibrosis for a diagnosis of steatohepatitis is likely too restrictive, because there is undoubtedly an earlier prefibrotic stage in steatohepatitis.[9] In daily practice, a surgical pathologist is frequently faced with this problem. It seems reasonable that the presence of more than occasional ballooned hepatocytes or rare Mallory-Denk bodies, and certainly sinusoidal fibrosis (in a properly performed trichrome stain, discussed later) should lead to a diagnosis of steatohepatitis and not just steatosis.

Grading Alcoholic Steatohepatitis

The grading of alcoholic steatohepatitis is of interest for studies of pathogenesis, natural history, and possible treatment modalities. Although there is currently no grading system validated specifically for alcoholic steatohepatitis, the most widely used system for grading NASH is also routinely applied to cases of alcoholic liver disease, because histologic distinction between these entities is often not possible.[9] In this system, grade 1, or mild, steatohepatitis is diagnosed when there is macrovesicular steatosis involving up to two-thirds of the parenchyma combined with occasional centrilobular hepatocyte ballooning and mild acute and chronic lobular inflammation. Portal inflammation is usually minimal in such cases. Grade 2, or moderate, steatohepatitis refers to cases with any degree of steatosis combined with obvious centrilobular ballooning degeneration, neutrophilic inflammation, and sinusoidal fibrosis (discussed later). Mild to moderate portal inflammation may also be present. Finally, when more than two-thirds of the parenchyma is involved by steatosis and there is marked ballooning degeneration, acute and chronic inflammation and sinusoidal fibrosis, a diagnosis of severe, or grade 3, steatohepatitis is appropriate. Cases of severe steatohepatitis often exhibit clusters of neutrophils in areas of ballooning degeneration, and some degree of portal inflammation is also usually present.

Although the degree of hepatocyte ballooning degeneration, inflammation, Mallory-Denk body formation, and fibrosis has been found to vary significantly between biopsies in NASH, comparable studies have not been performed in alcoholic liver disease.[10,11] However, it is likely that disease involvement in alcoholic steatohepatitis is also patchy. This variability in distribution could significantly affect grading and staging, and it may be responsible for discrepancies between sequential biopsies.

MACROVESICULAR STEATOSIS AND STEATOHEPATITIS IN OTHER CONDITIONS

Macrovesicular steatosis is a relatively common pathologic alteration occurring in up to 5% of liver biopsies. Steatohepatitis (rather than just simple steatosis) can also occur in conditions other than alcoholic liver disease and NASH; perhaps the best known of these conditions is amiodarone toxicity.[12] Ballooned hepatocytes containing Mallory-Denk bodies are quite prominent in amiodarone toxicity, whereas the degree of steatosis is quite mild (or absent). The presence of phospholipidosis by electron microscopy would confirm a diagnosis of amiodarone toxicity.[13] Chronic administration of the drug can result in the development of fibrosis with the same centrilobular predominance seen in alcoholic steatohepatitis. Improvement in the histologic appearance can occur with discontinuation of the drug, but it can take many months because of the long half-life of the metabolites. Tamoxifen has also been documented to cause simple steatosis and steatohepatitis.[14] Steatosis or steatohepatitis can occur as an early finding in Wilson disease, particularly in children and teenagers. If a patient happens to also abuse alcohol (or be obese), a diagnosis of Wilson disease might not be considered. All of these conditions should be kept in mind as alternative or concurrent diagnoses in patients exhibiting histologic features of alcoholic liver disease.

DISTINCTION BETWEEN ALCOHOLIC AND NONALCOHOLIC FATTY LIVER DISEASE

Although macrovesicular steatosis and steatohepatitis are seen in several conditions, the pathologic features of NASH most closely resemble those of alcoholic liver disease, and distinction between these two forms of steatohepatitis is generally not possible in an individual patient.[15,16] Studies do suggest that the degree of hepatocellular injury, inflammation, and fibrosis tends to be greater in alcoholics, but there is considerable overlap.[17,18] Additionally, patients with a history of significant alcohol consumption may also be obese and/or diabetic, in which case it may be impossible to determine the degree to which each etiologic factor is contributing to the patient's fatty liver disease. That said, certain patterns of injury associated with steatohepatitis have mainly been described in alcoholic liver disease. These conditions include cholestatic liver disease mimicking extrahepatic biliary obstruction, alcoholic foamy degeneration, and sclerosing hyaline necrosis, which are discussed in detail next.

Cholestatic Alcoholic Liver Disease Mimicking Extrahepatic Biliary Obstruction

A specific clinicopathologic pattern of alcoholic liver disease is recognized that closely simulates extrahepatic biliary obstruction.[19] The patients are often markedly jaundiced, with significantly elevated serum total bilirubin and alkaline phosphatase. Biopsies in these patients reveal edematous portal tracts with significant bile ductular proliferation and portal neutrophilic infiltrates. Prominent hepatocellular and canalicular cholestasis is also present (**Fig. 9**). Knowledge of this peculiar form of alcoholic liver disease allows avoidance of endoscopic retrograde cholangiopancreatography

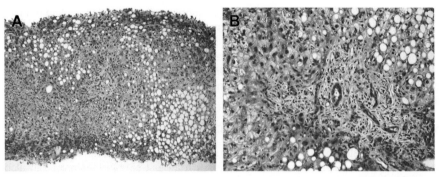

Fig. 9. Cholestatic alcoholic steatohepatitis. (*A*) The low-power view demonstrated canalicular cholestasis and a portal bile ductular reaction in addition to the typical features of steatohepatitis. (*B*) The high-power view of the portal tract reveals portal edema and ductular proliferation, further mimicking mechanical biliary obstruction (hematoxylin-eosin, original magnifications ×40 [*A*] and ×100 [*B*]).

(or exploratory laparotomy), which can carry a significant risk of morbidity in this patient population.[20] This pattern of cholestatic liver injury has not been documented in patients with NASH.[9]

Alcoholic Foamy Degeneration

In other jaundiced patients with alcoholism, particularly those with acute alcohol intoxication, a liver biopsy may reveal marked centrilobular microvesicular steatosis, a pattern that has been termed "alcoholic foamy degeneration." The hepatocytes in this condition are swollen and filled with small droplets of lipid, which do not displace the nucleus peripherally (**Fig. 10**). Megamitochondria are also often prominent in the foam-filled hepatocytes. Canalicular cholestasis is usually evident, but macrovesicular steatosis and neutrophilic infiltration are typically absent. These changes usually resolve within a few weeks of cessation of alcohol consumption, although

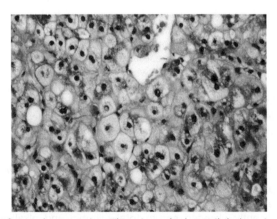

Fig. 10. Alcoholic foamy degeneration. There is marked centrilobular microvesicular steatosis, and a few scattered hepatocytes exhibiting macrovesicular steatosis. The figure highlights the central placement of the nucleus in the hepatocytes affected by microvesicular steatosis. Note also the presence of canalicular cholestasis (hematoxylin-eosin, original magnification ×200).

macrovesicular steatosis is often present in subsequent biopsies.[21,22] This form of liver damage also does not occur in patients with NASH.[9]

Sclerosing Hyaline Necrosis

Sclerosing hyaline necrosis represents a severe form of alcoholic steatohepatitis in which there is significant necrosis or dropout of centrilobular hepatocytes, with replacement by confluent fibrosis (**Fig. 11**). The sinusoidal strands of fibrosis also become very thick, and central veins are often occluded by fibrosis (phlebosclerosis or veno-occlusive like change).[23] Identification of sclerosing hyaline necrosis is important, because it has a poor prognosis and often leads to the development of significant portal hypertension and ascites.[24] The presence of sclerosing hyaline necrosis implicates alcohol as the main etiologic agent contributing to the patient's liver disease, because this condition is not typically seen in patients with NASH.[9]

FIBROSIS IN ALCOHOLIC LIVER DISEASE

Fibrosis beginning at the central vein (terminal hepatic venule) and extending into the lobules along the sinusoids is highly characteristic of steatohepatitis and is rarely seen in other conditions. The extension of fibrosis along the sinusoids, termed sinusoidal, perisinusoidal, or pericellular fibrosis, usually progresses radially, producing a cobweb, chicken wire, or maple leaf pattern. Sinusoidal fibrosis is difficult to detect on routine hematoxylin and eosin–stained sections, but a trichrome stain highlights the delicate sinusoidal collagen fibers in blue (**Fig. 12**). With disease progression, bands of fibrosis form between central veins (central-central bridging fibrosis) (**Fig. 13**) and between central veins and portal tracts (central-portal bridging fibrosis) (**Fig. 14**). Portal-portal bridging fibrosis may also be seen. Cirrhosis can be diagnosed when regenerative nodules of parenchyma are completely encircled by bands of fibrosis (**Fig. 15**). In alcoholic steatohepatitis, the cirrhosis that develops is of micronodular type, meaning that the individual regenerative nodules are smaller in size than hepatic lobules.

Attempts to identify histologic features that are predictive of fibrosis development in alcoholic liver disease have had limited success. Iron deposition, which is often seen in liver biopsies from patients with alcoholic liver disease and can be visualized using a

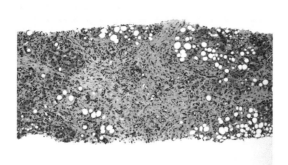

Fig. 11. Central hyaline necrosis. The centrilobular area exhibits confluent fibrosis with complete obliteration of the central vein (terminal hepatic venule) (hematoxylin-eosin, original magnification ×40).

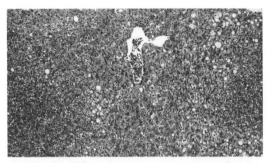

Fig. 12. Centrilobular fibrosis. This trichrome stain highlights the presence of delicate strands of pericellular fibrosis producing a characteristic "cobweb" pattern (trichrome, original magnification ×40).

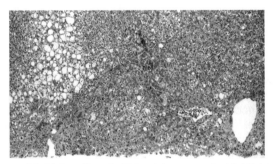

Fig. 13. Central-central bridging fibrosis. This trichrome stain highlights the presence of fibrosis linking adjacent central veins (trichrome, original magnification ×40).

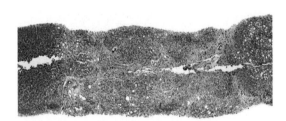

Fig. 14. Central-central and central-portal fibrosis. This trichrome stain highlights extensive bridging fibrosis resulting in early cirrhosis (trichrome, original magnification ×20).

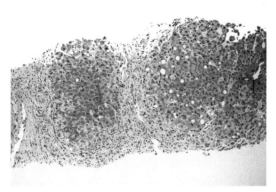

Fig. 15. Micronodular cirrhosis. This trichrome stain confirms the presence of small regenerative nodules of parenchyma that are completely encircled by bands of fibrosis, diagnostic of cirrhosis (trichrome, original magnification ×20).

Prussian blue stain, has been shown to be an independent risk factor for fibrosis development in patients with alcoholism.[25] Given the high frequency of cirrhosis in patients with hereditary hemochromatosis, the association between iron deposition and fibrosis in alcoholic liver disease is not surprising. Although less well-established, the presence of megamitochondria, which appear as large, round to needle-shaped, eosinophilic bodies and are often seen in patients with alcoholic liver disease, was also found to be predictive of fibrosis development in one study.[26] The recent discovery that a polymorphism in the patatin-like phospholipase domain-containing-3 gene is strongly associated with the development of fibrosis and cirrhosis in alcoholic liver disease has piqued new interest in the impact of genetic susceptibility on disease progression.[27,28] The relationship between the morphologic features of alcoholic liver disease and these emerging genetic risk factors has not yet been extensively investigated.

Although fibrosis was once considered an irreversible process, regression of fibrosis is now well-established in many forms of chronic liver injury. Conversion from micronodular to macronodular cirrhosis via resorption of fibrous septae is commonly seen in patients with alcoholic liver disease who undergo liver transplantation following months of abstinence (**Fig. 16**). Resorption of sinusoidal collagen fibers also likely occurs in alcoholic liver disease, because sinusoidal fibrosis is often no longer evident in explanted livers from abstinent patients with alcoholic liver disease.[29]

Staging Fibrosis

Accurate reporting of fibrosis in cases of alcoholic liver disease is important for clinical management and prognostic purposes. As with grading, a separate system for staging has not been validated in alcoholic steatohepatitis, but the staging system developed for NASH is frequently used.[9] In this system, the presence of focal or extensive sinusoidal fibrosis constitutes stage 1 fibrosis, and such fibrosis is usually evident in the subsequent stages of disease. Once focal or extensive periportal fibrosis develops, stage 2 fibrosis is diagnosed. If central-central, central-portal, or portal-portal bridging fibrosis is present, the stage increases to stage 3. Finally, when bridging fibrosis is accompanied by hepatocyte regeneration and nodule formation, a diagnosis of stage

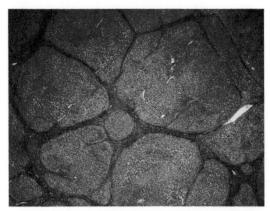

Fig. 16. Evolution to macronodular cirrhosis. This trichrome stain illustrates the conversion of micronodular cirrhosis to macronodular cirrhosis in a patient with alcoholic steatohepatitis who has had prolonged alcohol abstinence. Some of the fibrous septae are being remodeled and smaller nodules have coalesced to form larger nodules. There is no evidence of residual active steatohepatitis (trichrome, original magnification ×40).

4 fibrosis, or cirrhosis, is rendered. The development of fibrosis in chronic viral and autoimmune hepatitis is strictly portal based and therefore the systems used to stage fibrosis in chronic hepatitis (eg, the Batts-Ludwig system) are not useful in cases of steatohepatitis and should not be used.

Alcoholic Cirrhosis and Hepatocellular Carcinoma

Alcoholic cirrhosis is classically micronodular, with persistence of sinusoidal fibrosis often evident in trichrome-stained sections. Evolution to a macronodular pattern is common with prolonged abstinence from ethanol, and most native livers removed at the time of transplantation exhibit either a mixed micronodular and macronodular or pure macronodular pattern.[29,30] Once cirrhosis is present, the risk of hepatocellular carcinoma is estimated at 5% to 15%, making alcoholic cirrhosis one of the most common settings for the development of hepatocellular carcinoma in the United States.[31,32] The morphologic features of hepatocellular carcinoma in patients with alcoholic cirrhosis are similar to those seen in other settings, and further discussion of these features is beyond the scope of this review.

ALCOHOLIC HEPATITIS HISTOLOGIC SCORE

Recently, a new histologic scoring system for predicting short-term mortality in patients with alcoholic liver disease was proposed based on the results of a large, multicenter study.[33] In this study, multivariate logistic regression analysis identified extensive fibrosis, lack of neutrophilic inflammation, presence of cholestasis, and absence of megamitochondria as independent predictors of 90-day mortality. Based on these findings, an Alcoholic Hepatitis Histologic Score was developed (**Table 1**). A total score of 0 to 3 signifies a low risk of short-term mortality, a score of 4 to 5 indicates an intermediate risk of 90-day mortality, and a score of 6 to 9 predicts a high risk of death within 90 days. Although this system underwent external validation as part of the initial study, further assessment of the reproducibility and utility of this scoring system is necessary before its routine use can be recommended.

Table 1
Alcoholic Hepatitis Histologic Score point distribution

Component		Points
Stage of fibrosis	No fibrosis or portal fibrosis	0
	Expansive fibrosis	0
	Bridging fibrosis or cirrhosis	+3
Degree of neutrophil infiltration	None	+2
	Severe	0
Pattern of cholestasis	None	0
	Hepatocellular only	0
	Canalicular/ductular	+1
	Hepatocellular plus canalicular/ductular	+2
Megamitochondria	None	+2
	Present	0

Adapted from Altamirano J, Miquel R, Katoonizadeh A, et al. A histologic scoring system for prognosis of patients with alcoholic hepatitis. Gastroenterology 2014;146(5):1231–9.e1–6.

COMORBID CONDITIONS IN ALCOHOLIC LIVER DISEASE

Although alcoholic liver disease can frequently be diagnosed on clinical grounds alone, a common reason to obtain a liver biopsy in patients with alcohol abuse is to identify comorbidities that may be contributing to the patient's liver disease. Such conditions are not uncommon; up to 20% of patients with alcoholic liver disease are reported to have an additional source of liver injury.[34] The discovery of coexistent etiologies for liver disease has important therapeutic implications. Furthermore, several of the commonly detected liver diseases have morphologic features that overlap with those of alcoholic liver disease. The pathologist should be aware of such conditions, and the threshold for their clinical exclusion should be low. Liver diseases of particular importance in this regard include α_1-antitrypsin (A1AT) deficiency, hemochromatosis, and hepatitis C infection.

Cytoplasmic accumulation of A1AT globules is frequently encountered in alcoholic liver disease. These globules appear as round, brightly eosinophilic intracytoplasmic inclusions that stain intensely with periodic acid–Schiff with diastase (**Fig. 17**). Although the distribution of these globules may be more diffuse in alcoholic liver disease than the typical periportal pattern seen in hereditary A1AT deficiency, measurement of the serum A1AT level or genotype analysis is recommended in cases where such globules are identified. Given the increased prevalence of hereditary A1AT deficiency seen in explanted livers from patients with alcoholism, the co-occurrence of these conditions likely hastens the progression of alcoholic liver disease.[32]

Iron stores are frequently increased in patients with alcoholic liver disease, and the presence of hepatocellular iron deposition likely contributes to liver injury and the risk of disease progression and fibrosis.[35] However, many patients with hereditary iron storage disorders, such as hereditary hemochromatosis, also consume significant quantities of alcohol. Although the degree of iron deposition is typically greater in hereditary hemochromatosis than in alcoholic liver disease alone, the coexistence of a hereditary iron storage condition must always be considered in patients with increased hepatic iron detected by Prussian blue stain.[31] Quantitative assessment of liver iron stores using biochemical methods is helpful in differentiating between hereditary and secondary causes of iron deposition, but genetic testing may also be necessary.

The prevalence of hepatitis C infection is increased in patients with chronic alcohol abuse, and the coexistence of these conditions has a synergistic effect on the progression of liver disease and the risk of hepatocellular carcinoma.[32,35–37] Although inflammation and fibrosis are morphologic manifestations of both diseases, there are several histologic features distinct to each condition. Dense portal lymphocytic inflammation with extension into the adjacent parenchyma (interface activity) signifies active involvement by hepatitis C, whereas the presence of neutrophils and ballooned hepatocytes in the lobules indicates a component of alcoholic steatohepatitis (**Fig. 18**). Although chronic hepatitis C infection results in portal-based fibrosis, alcohol-related fibrosis is predominantly centrilobular, at least in its initial stages. In some cases, the severity of these features can help identify the etiologic agent responsible for a patient's worsening liver function. However, the precise contribution of each condition is often impossible to determine, and both diseases usually play a role in the progression of liver disease.

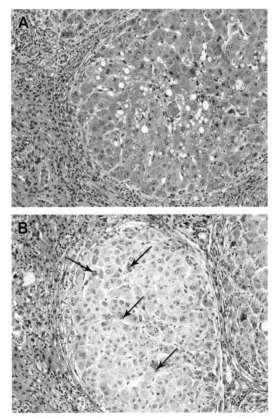

Fig. 17. Cirrhosis caused by alcoholic steatohepatitis with superimposed α_1-antitrypsin deficiency. (*A*) The hematoxylin and eosin section demonstrates micronodular cirrhosis with mild ongoing steatohepatitis. (*B*) In the periodic acid–Schiff with diastase stained section the magenta-colored globules (*arrows*) of α_1-antitrypsin can be seen in the periseptal hepatocytes ([*A*] hematoxylin-eosin and [*B*] periodic acid-Schiff with diastase, original magnification ×100).

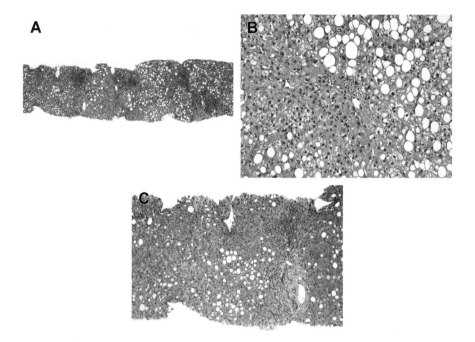

Fig. 18. Alcoholic steatohepatitis with superimposed chronic hepatitis C virus (HCV) hepatitis. (A) The low-power view demonstrates dense portal lymphocytic infiltrates caused by the chronic HCV infection (hematoxylin-eosin, original magnification ×20). Portal tract inflammation of this severity is not consistent with alcoholic steatohepatitis alone. (B) The higher power view demonstrates mild steatosis and scattered ballooned hepatocytes, consistent with superimposed steatohepatitis (hematoxylin-eosin, original magnification ×100). (C) The trichrome stain reveals portal and centrilobular fibrosis. Alcoholic steatohepatitis and chronic HCV hepatitis can result in portal fibrosis, but only steatohepatitis causes centrilobular fibrosis (trichrome, original magnification ×40).

SUMMARY

The pathologic diagnosis of alcoholic liver disease requires a clinical history of significant alcohol use combined with certain histologic findings, including macrovesicular steatosis, hepatocellular ballooning degeneration, Mallory-Denk bodies, neutrophilic infiltration, and/or sinusoidal fibrosis. However, the morphology of alcoholic liver disease varies considerably between patients, and many of the microscopic findings overlap significantly with those seen in other forms of liver injury (especially NASH). Therefore, awareness of the full range of histologic features of alcoholic liver disease and consideration of comorbid conditions is crucial when evaluating liver specimens from patients with alcoholism.

REFERENCES

1. Budd G. Diseases of the liver. 3rd edition. London: John Churchill; 1857.
2. French SW, Nash J, Shitabata P, et al. Pathology of alcoholic liver disease. Semin Liver Dis 1993;13:154–69.
3. Mallory FB. Cirrhosis of the liver, five different types of lesions from which it may arise. Bull Johns Hopkins Hosp 1911;22:69–74.

4. Ludwig J, Viggiano TR, McGill DB, et al. Non-alcoholic steatohepatitis. Mayo Clinic experience with a hitherto unnamed disease. Mayo Clin Proc 1980;55:434–8.
5. Jensen K, Gluud C. The Mallory body: morphological, clinical and experimental studies (Part 1 of a literature survey). Hepatology 1994;20:1061–77.
6. Jensen K, Gluud C. The Mallory body: theories on development and pathological significance (Part 2 of a literature survey). Hepatology 1994;20:1330–42.
7. Banner BF, Savas L, Zivny J, et al. Ubiquitin as a marker of cell injury in nonalcoholic steatohepatitis. Am J Clin Pathol 2000;114:860–6.
8. Colombat M, Charlotte F, Ratziu V, et al. Portal lymphocytic infiltrate in alcoholic liver disease. Hum Pathol 2002;33(12):1170–4.
9. Brunt EM. Nonalcoholic steatohepatitis: definition and pathology. Semin Liver Dis 2001;21:3–16.
10. Goldstein NS, Hastah F, Galan MV, et al. Fibrosis heterogeneity in non-alcoholic steatohepatitis and hepatitis C virus needle core biopsy specimens. Am J Clin Pathol 2005;123:382–7.
11. Ratziu V, Charlotte F, Heurtier A, et al. Sampling variability of liver biopsy in nonalcoholic liver disease. Gastroenterology 2005;128:1898–906.
12. Stravitz RT, Sanyal AJ. Drug-induced steatohepatitis. Clin Liver Dis 2003;7:435–51.
13. Lewis JH, Ranard RC, Caruso A, et al. Amiodarone hepatotoxicity: prevalence and clinicopathologic correlations among 104 patients. Hepatology 1989;9:679–85.
14. Hamada N, Ogawa Y, Saibara T, et al. Toremifene-induced fatty liver and NASH in breast cancer patients with breast-conservation treatment. Int J Oncol 2000;17: 1119–23.
15. Lee RG. Nonalcoholic steatohepatitis: a study of 49 patients. Hum Pathol 1989; 20:594–9.
16. Wanless IR, Lentz JS. Fatty liver hepatitis (steatohepatitis) and obesity: an autopsy study with analysis of risk factors. Hepatology 1990;12:1106–10.
17. Itoh S, Yougel T, Kawagoe K, et al. Comparison between nonalcoholic steatohepatitis and alcoholic hepatitis. Am J Gastroenterol 1987;82:650–4.
18. Pinto HC, Baptista A, Camilo ME, et al. Nonalcoholic steatohepatitis. Clinicopathological comparison with alcoholic hepatitis in ambulatory and hospitalized patients. Dig Dis Sci 1996;41:172–9.
19. Phillips GB, Davidson CS. Liver disease of the chronic alcoholic simulating extrahepatic biliary obstruction. Gastroenterology 1957;33:236–44.
20. Nissenbaum M, Chedid A, Mendenhall C, et al. Prognostic significance of cholestatic alcoholic hepatitis. Dig Dis Sci 1990;35:891–6.
21. Uchida T, Kao H, Quispe-Sjogren M, et al. Alcoholic foamy degeneration: a pattern of acute alcoholic injury of the liver. Gastroenterology 1983;84:683–92.
22. Lefkowitch JH. Morphology of alcoholic liver disease. Clin Liver Dis 2005;9: 37–53.
23. Goodman ZD, Ishak KG. Occlusive venous lesions in alcoholic liver disease. A study of 200 cases. Gastroenterology 1982;83:786–96.
24. Fleming KA, McGee JO. Alcohol induced liver disease. J Clin Pathol 1984;37(7): 721–33.
25. Raynard B, Balian A, Fallik D, et al. Risk factors of fibrosis in alcohol-induced liver disease. Hepatology 2002;35:635–8.
26. Teli MR, Day CP, Burt AD, et al. Determinants of progression to cirrhosis or fibrosis in pure alcoholic fatty liver. Lancet 1995;346(8981):987–90.
27. Trépo E, Gustot T, Degré D, et al. Common polymorphism in the PNPLA3/adiponutrin gene confers higher risk of cirrhosis and liver damage in alcoholic liver disease. J Hepatol 2011;55(4):906–12.

28. Burza MA, Molinaro A, Attilia ML, et al. PNPLA3 I148M (rs738409) genetic variant and age at onset of at-risk alcohol consumption are independent risk factors for alcoholic cirrhosis. Liver Int 2014;34(4):514–20.
29. Wanless IR, Nakashima E, Sherman M. Regression of human cirrhosis. Morphologic features and the genesis of incomplete septal cirrhosis. Arch Pathol Lab Med 2000;124(11):1599–607.
30. Fauerholdt L, Schlichting P, Christensen E, et al. Conversion of micronodular cirrhosis into macronodular cirrhosis. Hepatology 1983;3:928–31.
31. Ishak KG, Zimmerman HJ, Ray MB. Alcoholic liver disease: pathologic, pathogenetic and clinical aspects. Alcohol Clin Exp Res 1991;15(1):45–66.
32. Yip WW, Burt AD. Alcoholic liver disease. Semin Diagn Pathol 2006;23(3–4): 149–60.
33. Altamirano J, Miquel R, Katoonizadeh A, et al. A histologic scoring system for prognosis of patients with alcoholic hepatitis. Gastroenterology 2014;146(5): 1231–9.e1–6.
34. Sakhuja P. Pathology of alcoholic liver disease, can it be differentiated from nonalcoholic steatohepatitis? World J Gastroenterol 2014;20(44):16474–9.
35. Safdar K, Schiff ER. Alcohol and hepatitis C. Semin Liver Dis 2004;24(3):305–15.
36. Mueller S, Millonig G, Seitz HK. Alcoholic liver disease and hepatitis C: a frequently underestimated combination. World J Gastroenterol 2009;15(28):3462–71.
37. Shoreibah M, Anand BS, Singal AK. Alcoholic hepatitis and concomitant hepatitis C virus infection. World J Gastroenterol 2014;20(34):11929–34.

Prognosis and Prognostic Scoring Models for Alcoholic Liver Disease and Acute Alcoholic Hepatitis

CrossMark

Pierre M. Gholam, MD

KEYWORDS

- Maddrey score • GAHS • MELD • Discriminant function • ABIC

KEY POINTS

- A discriminant function greater than or equal to 32 denotes increased mortality at 30 and 90 days.
- Acute alcoholic hepatitis prognostic scores perform better at predicting patients likely to achieve short-term survival rather than those at high risk of death.
- Combining prognostic factors may improve the ability to identify patients at high risk of death and nonresponders to medical therapy.

INTRODUCTION

Prognostic scoring models are relevant in conditions where associated morbidity and mortality are high. It is therefore not surprising that several of these exist for acute alcoholic hepatitis (AAH). The main value of these scores is to provide validated risk assessment at baseline, which allows for prognostication and follow-up information on response to a specific therapy or to assess for spontaneous improvement in cases when treatment is declined or not indicated. Although multiple randomized controlled clinical trials have used one or more of these scores for entry and outcome purposes, they all present some limitations, which are highlighted later. This article focuses on scores that are widely used in clinical practice and have some degree of specificity to liver disease. The most commonly used scoring systems are discussed here in detail (**Table 1**). Other scores that predict the outcome of serious illness, such as the Acute Physiology and Chronic Health Evaluation II score, are not discussed here.[1]

The author has nothing to disclose.
Liver Center of Excellence, Digestive Health Institute, University Hospitals Case Medical Center, 11100 Euclid Avenue, WRN5066, Cleveland Heights, OH 44104, USA
E-mail address: Pierre.Gholam@case.edu

Clin Liver Dis 20 (2016) 491–497
http://dx.doi.org/10.1016/j.cld.2016.02.007
1089-3261/16/$ – see front matter © 2016 Elsevier Inc. All rights reserved.

Table 1
Prognostic clinical scores of alcoholic hepatitis

Score	Calculation Formula				Severe Disease Indicator
Maddrey discriminant function	4.6 × [patient's prothrombin time (seconds) − control prothrombin time (seconds)] + bilirubin (mg/dL)				≥32
Model for end-stage liver disease	$3.8 \times \log_e$ bilirubin (mg/dL) + $11.2 \times \log_e$ INR + $9.6 \times \log_e$ creatinine (mg/dL) + 6.4				≥21
Glasgow alcoholic hepatitis score		1	2	3	≥9
	Age (y)	<50	≥50	—	
	WCC (10^9/L)	<15	≥15	—	
	Urea (mmol/L)	<5	≥5	—	
	PT ratio	<1.5	1.5–2.0	>2.0	
	Bilirubin (μmol/L)	<125	125–250	>250	
	Sum the points assigned for each of the 5 factors				
ABIC (age, serum bilirubin, INR, and serum creatinine)	Age (y) × 0.1 + bilirubin (mg/dL) × 0.08 + creatinine (mg/dL) × 0.3 + INR × 0.8				>9
Lille score	(Exp[−R]/[1 + Exp(−R)]), where R = 3.19− 0.101 × age (y) + 0.147 × albumin (g/L) + 0.0165 × change in bilirubin (total bilirubin at Day 0 μmol/L − total bilirubin at Day 7 in μmol/L) − 0.206 × renal insufficiency (0 or 1) − 0.0065 × total bilirubin at Day 0 (μmol/L) − 0.0096 × prothrombin time (seconds) Renal insufficiency is rated as 1 if creatinine level at Day 0 is ≥1.3 mg/dL, and as 0 if creatinine level is <1.3 mg/dL				>0.45

Abbreviations: INR, international normalized ratio; PT, prothrombin time; WCC, white blood cell count.

MODIFIED DISCRIMINANT FUNCTION OR MADDREY SCORE

The realization that biochemical parameters reflecting liver injury and synthetic function can predict short-term mortality based on experience with early clinical trials led to the development of the original discriminant function (DF), which was later slightly modified and remains extensively used today.[2,3] The formula is as follows:

4.6 × [Protime patient − control (in seconds)] + total bilirubin (mg/dL)

Perhaps the most valuable information provided by DF is its ability to predict 28-day mortality in the setting of severe alcoholic hepatitis (AH). Although different studies have yielded somewhat variable results, one large randomized controlled trial showed that a DF greater than or equal to 32 was associated with a 68% 28-day survival in placebo-treated patients, whereas those with a score less than 32 had a survival of 93%.[3] A baseline DF greater than 32 has been shown to be associated with a markedly reduced survival and thus has been used to define "severe" AH. A score lower than 32 is generally accepted to denote a more favorable short-term prognosis with the notable exception of patients who develop hepatic encephalopathy. This has led to DF greater than 32 being widely used as an entry criterion for clinical trials exploring the efficacy of new and existing therapies.[4,5] Other studies have suggested that mortality in patients with DF less than 32 is not trivial and may exclude patients who could benefit from therapy or participation in clinical trials.[6]

Despite the advent of other prognostic and severity scores, DF remains widely used in clinical practice. Perhaps the biggest shortcoming of DF is its static nature, which lacks validation over time because biochemical parameters evolve depending on spontaneous improvement, response to therapy, or lack thereof. Recent evidence suggests that combining DF with other models that address these issues may accurately predict patient outcomes better than any of them by itself (discussed later).[7]

The other practical issue is that calculation of DF requires the absolute value of the prothrombin time, which can vary significantly depending on the assays used in different laboratories or countries and may create significant variation in scores.[8] Although some suggestions have been made to mitigate this including use of the geometric mean of the prothrombin time, there is currently no widely accepted consensus on how to address this issue.

GLASGOW ALCOHOLIC HEPATITIS SCORE

Glasgow alcoholic hepatitis score (GAHS) is a more recent attempt to provide a dynamic assessment of mortality risk and prognosis using readily available biochemical parameters and their evolution over time.[9] GAHS is derived from the following variables: age, Day 1 serum bilirubin, Day 1 blood urea, Day 6 to 9 serum bilirubin, prothrombin time, and peripheral blood white blood cell count (**Table 2**).

GAHS scores range from 5 to 12. For patients with a GAHS greater than or equal to 9, the 28-day survival for untreated and corticosteroid-treated patients was 52% and 78% ($P = .002$), and 84-day survival was 38% and 59% ($P = .02$), respectively, indicating more severe disease and potentially identifying patients who may benefit from therapy among those with DF greater than 32.[10] Baseline GAHS determination had an overall accuracy of 81% when predicting 28-day outcome.[11] In contrast, DF had an overall accuracy of 49% based on validation study data. Day 6 to 9 data also seem to predict 84-day mortality accurately. GAHS may compare favorably with the ABIC score (discussed next). Although GAHS has not been frequently used for entry purposes in clinical trials, it seemed to perform well as a predictor of poor prognosis in a recent large randomized clinical trial.[12]

Table 2 The Glasgow alcoholic hepatitis score			
Factor	1	2	3
Age	<50	≥50	—
WCC (10^9/L)	<15	≥15	—
Urea (mmol/L)	<5	≥5	—
PT ratio	<1.5	1.5–2.0	>2.0
Bilirubin (μmol/L)	<125	125–250	>250

Abbreviations: PT, prothrombin time; WCC, white blood cell count.

Data from Forrest EH, Evans CD, Stewart S, et al. Analysis of factors predictive of mortality in alcoholic hepatitis and derivation and validation of the Glasgow alcoholic hepatitis score. Gut 2005;54(8):1174–79.

AGE, SERUM BILIRUBIN, INTERNATIONAL NORMALIZED RATIO AND CREATININE SCORE

ABIC is an acronym for Age, serum Bilirubin, International normalized ratio (INR), and Creatinine.[13] The formula was derived from a cohort of patients with biopsy-proven AAH then validated and is as follows:

(Age × 0.1) + (total bilirubin (mg/dL) × 0.08) + (serum creatinine (mg/dL) × 0.3) + (INR × 0.8)

ABIC cutoff values of less than or equal to 6.71, 6.71 to 9, and greater than 9.0 categorize patients into low, intermediate, and high risk of 90-day death (100%, 70%, and 25% of survival, respectively). The score compares well with others listed in this article, although one limitation that it shares with many of them is that its negative predictive value is significantly better than its positive predictive value for death making it better at identifying patients at low rather than high risk for death.[14,15]

LILLE SCORE

The paucity of effective therapies for AAH and the need for early identification of patients with severe AH (defined as DF ≥32) not responding to corticosteroids led to the development of the Lille score.[16] Six reproducible variables (age, renal insufficiency, albumin, prothrombin time, bilirubin, and evolution of bilirubin at Day 7) were incorporated into the model. A Lille score calculator is available online (http://www.lillemodel.com/score.asp), which aids with the generation of a score derivation from a complex algorithm. Another version that incorporates INR instead of prothrombin time is also available. It is advised to use prealbumin infusion laboratory values to avoid artificial inflation of this parameter when generating a score. A significant advantage of the Lille score is a dynamic component in the form of bilirubin evolution, which is the single most heavily weighted component and has good accuracy for predicting 6-month mortality.[17]

Patients with a Lille score higher than 0.45 had a 25% 6-month survival versus 85% for others (**Fig. 1**). This cutoff was able to identify approximately 75% of the observed

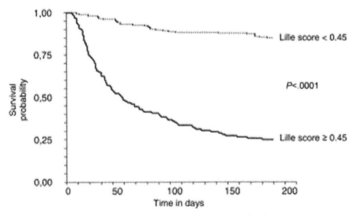

Fig. 1. Kaplan-Meier survival analysis according to 0.45 cutoff of the Lille model. (*From* Louvet A, Naveau S, Abdelnour M, et al. The Lille model: a new tool for therapeutic strategy in patients with severe alcoholic hepatitis treated with steroids. Hepatology 2007;45(6): 1352; with permission.)

deaths during cohort validation. A Lille score of greater than 0.45 also suggests that a patient with AH is not responding to steroids. This allows termination of this therapy.

In comparison with other available prognostic models, the Lille score showed a higher area under the curve suggesting better prediction of 6-month survival (**Fig. 2**).[16]

The Lille score has since been applied in a variety of settings including to determine nonresponse to medical therapies in patients deemed candidates for liver transplantation, and meta-analyses of patient data to assess short-term survival in response to different therapies.[18–22]

MODEL FOR END-STAGE LIVER DISEASE

Since its development as a prognostic tool for mortality from transjugular intrahepatic portosystemic hunting, model for end-stage liver disease (MELD) has become the most widely used scoring system in the setting of advanced liver disease with applications ranging from assigning liver transplant organ allocation priority to assessing the risk of morbidity and mortality from surgery in patients with cirrhosis.[23–25] As a robust predictor of mortality from liver disease, it is not surprising that MELD performs well in the setting of AH. Although early studies suggested that MELD may be equivalent to DF in its ability to predict 30- and 90-day mortality, some have suggested it may offer an advantage, whereas others came to different conclusions.[26–28]

The MELD formula is as follows:

$$3.78 \times \ln[\text{total bilirubin (mg/dL)}] + 11.2 \times \ln[\text{INR}] + 9.57 \times \ln[\text{serum creatinine (mg/dL)}] + 6.43$$

MELD suffers from some of the same limitations of other prognostic scores in that it seems to identify patients at low risk of short-term mortality rather than those at highest risk. Although there is no universally accepted cut-off for a MELD value above which mortality is increased, a value of 18 has been quoted in expert reviews, whereas a MELD of 21 was found to have 75% sensitivity and specificity in predicting 90-day mortality.[26,29] A change in MELD over time may also predict poorer outcomes and higher in-hospital mortality.[27]

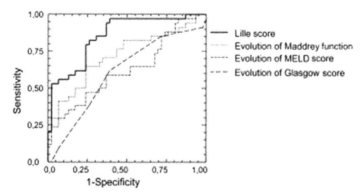

Fig. 2. Receiver operating characteristic curves for survival at 6 months in the validation cohort as determined by the Lille model versus the evolution of the Maddrey function (*P* = .03), the MELD score (*P* = .01), the Glasgow score (*P* = .0008), and the Child-Pugh score (*P* = .003). (*From* Louvet A, Naveau S, Abdelnour M, et al. The Lille model: a new tool for therapeutic strategy in patients with severe alcoholic hepatitis treated with steroids. Hepatology 2007;45(6):1352; with permission.)

COMBINING PROGNOSTIC MODELS

The currently used models for predicting AH prognosis each have benefits and disadvantages. Louvet and colleagues[7] performed a study in 2015 looking at the utility of combining prognostic models to improve outcome prediction. They compared DF + Lille versus MELD + Lille versus ABIC + Lille. Looking at 2- and 6-month mortality rates, they found that MELD + Lille model was the best at predicting mortality in patients with severe AH.

SUMMARY

The DF remains the most widely used prognostic score in clinical practice for AH and DF greater than or equal to 32 has remained largely synonymous with severe disease. Most clinical trials continue to use this as the main entry criterion to identify patients who are at risk of death and may benefit from pharmacologic or other interventions. The ability to identify patients at high risk of death may be improved by combining results from static and dynamic scoring systems for liver disease compared with one model alone. As new experimental agents make their way to clinical trials, this will become a crucial issue in identifying the most appropriate study population.

REFERENCES

1. Duseja A, Choudhary NS, Gupta S, et al. APACHE II score is superior to SOFA, CTP and MELD in predicting the short-term mortality in patients with acute-on-chronic liver failure (ACLF). J Dig Dis 2013;14(9):484–90.
2. Maddrey WC, Boitnott JK, Bedine MS, et al. Corticosteroid therapy of alcoholic hepatitis. Gastroenterology 1978;75(2):193–9.
3. Carithers RL Jr, Herlong HF, Diehl AM, et al. Methylprednisolone therapy in patients with severe alcoholic hepatitis. A randomized multicenter trial. Ann Intern Med 1989;110(9):685–90.
4. Akriviadis E, Botla R, Briggs W, et al. Pentoxifylline improves short-term survival in severe acute alcoholic hepatitis: a double-blind, placebo-controlled trial. Gastroenterology 2000;119(6):1637–48.
5. Tilg H, Jalan R, Kaser A, et al. Anti-tumor necrosis factor-alpha monoclonal antibody therapy in severe alcoholic hepatitis. J Hepatol 2003;38(4):419–25.
6. Kulkarni K, Tran T, Medrano M, et al. The role of the discriminant factor in the assessment and treatment of alcoholic hepatitis. J Clin Gastroenterol 2004; 38(5):453–9.
7. Louvet A, Labreuche J, Artru F, et al. Combining data from liver disease scoring systems better predicts outcomes of patients with alcoholic hepatitis. Gastroenterology 2015;149(2):398–406 e398 [quiz: e316–397].
8. Tilg H, Kaser A. Predicting mortality by the Glasgow alcoholic hepatitis score: the long awaited progress? Gut 2005;54(8):1057–9.
9. Forrest EH, Evans CD, Stewart S, et al. Analysis of factors predictive of mortality in alcoholic hepatitis and derivation and validation of the Glasgow alcoholic hepatitis score. Gut 2005;54(8):1174–9.
10. Forrest EH, Morris AJ, Stewart S, et al. The Glasgow alcoholic hepatitis score identifies patients who may benefit from corticosteroids. Gut 2007;56(12):1743–6.
11. Forrest EH, Fisher NC, Singhal S, et al. Comparison of the Glasgow alcoholic hepatitis score and the ABIC score for the assessment of alcoholic hepatitis. Am J Gastroenterol 2010;105(3):701–2.

12. Thursz MR, Richardson P, Allison M, et al. Prednisolone or pentoxifylline for alcoholic hepatitis. N Engl J Med 2015;372(17):1619–28.
13. Dominguez M, Rincon D, Abraldes JG, et al. A new scoring system for prognostic stratification of patients with alcoholic hepatitis. Am J Gastroenterol 2008;103(11): 2747–56.
14. Sandahl TD, Jepsen P, Ott P, et al. Validation of prognostic scores for clinical use in patients with alcoholic hepatitis. Scand J Gastroenterol 2011;46(9):1127–32.
15. Papastergiou V, Tsochatzis EA, Pieri G, et al. Nine scoring models for short-term mortality in alcoholic hepatitis: cross-validation in a biopsy-proven cohort. Aliment Pharmacol Ther 2014;39(7):721–32.
16. Louvet A, Naveau S, Abdelnour M, et al. The Lille model: a new tool for therapeutic strategy in patients with severe alcoholic hepatitis treated with steroids. Hepatology 2007;45(6):1348–54.
17. Mathurin P, Abdelnour M, Ramond MJ, et al. Early change in bilirubin levels is an important prognostic factor in severe alcoholic hepatitis treated with prednisolone. Hepatology 2003;38(6):1363–9.
18. Mathurin P, O'Grady J, Carithers RL, et al. Corticosteroids improve short-term survival in patients with severe alcoholic hepatitis: meta-analysis of individual patient data. Gut 2011;60(2):255–60.
19. Sharma P, Kumar A, Sharma BC, et al. Infliximab monotherapy for severe alcoholic hepatitis and predictors of survival: an open label trial. J Hepatol 2009; 50(3):584–91.
20. Sidhu SS, Goyal O, Singla P, et al. Corticosteroid plus pentoxifylline is not better than corticosteroid alone for improving survival in severe alcoholic hepatitis (COPE trial). Dig Dis Sci 2012;57(6):1664–71.
21. Mathurin P, Louvet A, Duhamel A, et al. Prednisolone with vs without pentoxifylline and survival of patients with severe alcoholic hepatitis: a randomized clinical trial. JAMA 2013;310(10):1033–41.
22. Mathurin P, Moreno C, Samuel D, et al. Early liver transplantation for severe alcoholic hepatitis. N Engl J Med 2011;365(19):1790–800.
23. Kamath PS, Wiesner RH, Malinchoc M, et al. A model to predict survival in patients with end-stage liver disease. Hepatology 2001;33(2):464–70.
24. Wiesner R, Edwards E, Freeman R, et al. Model for end-stage liver disease (MELD) and allocation of donor livers. Gastroenterology 2003;124(1):91–6.
25. Teh SH, Nagorney DM, Stevens SR, et al. Risk factors for mortality after surgery in patients with cirrhosis. Gastroenterology 2007;132(4):1261–9.
26. Dunn W, Jamil LH, Brown LS, et al. MELD accurately predicts mortality in patients with alcoholic hepatitis. Hepatology 2005;41(2):353–8.
27. Srikureja W, Kyulo NL, Runyon BA, et al. MELD score is a better prognostic model than Child-Turcotte-Pugh score or Discriminant Function score in patients with alcoholic hepatitis. J Hepatol 2005;42(5):700–6.
28. Monsanto P, Almeida N, Lrias C, et al. Evaluation of MELD score and Maddrey discriminant function for mortality prediction in patients with alcoholic hepatitis. Hepatogastroenterology 2013;60(125):1089–94.
29. Singal AK, Kamath PS, Gores GJ, et al. Alcoholic hepatitis: current challenges and future directions. Clin Gastroenterol Hepatol 2014;12(4):555–64 [quiz: e531–552].

Acute Alcoholic Hepatitis, the Clinical Aspects

Mohannad F. Dugum, MD[a], Arthur J. McCullough, MD[b],*

KEYWORDS

- Alcoholic hepatitis • Alcoholic liver disease • Diagnosis • Clinical outcomes

KEY POINTS

- The incidence of alcoholic hepatitis varies and depends on the amount, duration, and patterns of alcohol consumption; most patients consume more than 100 g/d of alcohol.
- Risk factors include age, female gender, ethnicity, obesity, malnutrition, coexistent hepatitis C virus infection, and genetic susceptibility.
- Diagnosis is mostly clinical based on history, physical examination, and a number of laboratory derangements.
- Several scoring models have been developed to assess disease severity and guide therapeutic decisions.
- Natural history and long-term outcomes are variable and partly dependent on abstinence from alcohol use. Recidivism is a major obstacle to recovery.

INTRODUCTION

Alcohol is a socially accepted hepatotoxin and its use is common worldwide with geographic variability in consumption patterns driven in part by local cultures and habits. The health-related consequences of alcohol are immense and depend on a number of factors related to the patterns of alcohol consumption, as well as an individual's comorbidities and genetic predisposition to alcohol's pathophysiological effects. Alcoholic liver disease (ALD) is a leading cause of advanced liver disease and is the leading cause of death in adults who drink excessively. The majority of liver disease burden in Western countries is attributable to alcohol use.[1] An acute form of ALD, alcoholic hepatitis (AH) is regarded as a specific clinical entity characterized by

This work was supported in part by Grant U01AA021893 from the National Institute on Alcohol Abuse and Alcoholism to A.J. McCullough. M.F. Dugum has nothing to disclose.
[a] Division of Gastroenterology, Hepatology and Nutrition, University of Pittsburgh, 200 Lothrop Street, UPMC Presbyterian, M2, C-Wing, Pittsburgh, PA 15213, USA; [b] Department of Gastroenterology and Hepatology, Digestive Disease Institute, Cleveland Clinic, 9500 Euclid Avenue, A30, Cleveland, OH 44195, USA
* Corresponding author. Department of Gastroenterology and Hepatology, Digestive Disease Institute, Cleveland Clinic, 9500 Euclid Avenue, A30, Cleveland, OH 44195.
E-mail address: mcculla@ccf.org

rapid decompensation of hepatic function. The severity spectrum of AH is wide with disease ranging from a subclinical form with good short-term outcomes to severe acute illness associated with high mortality. Early detection of high-risk patients and prompt intervention are needed to improve outcomes in patients with AH and alleviate the health care burden associated with severe disease.

Prevalence of Alcoholic Hepatitis

The exact incidence and prevalence of AH remain unclear, because many patients have subclinical disease and are never diagnosed. One study reported the prevalence of AH in a cohort of 1604 alcoholics to be approximately 20% based on liver biopsy data.[2] According to a study using the National Inpatient Sample, AH accounted for 56,809 hospitalizations in the United States in 2007 (0.71% of all hospitalizations). The mean age of admitted patients was 53 years, 75% of them were males, and the overall inpatient mortality was 6.8%. Acute renal failure, infections, hepatic encephalopathy, coagulopathy, and ascites were strongly associated with mortality.[3]

Patterns of Alcohol Intake Leading to Alcoholic Hepatitis

AH has been linked with excessive alcohol drinking over a prolonged period of time (typically >2 decades). However, it is now recognized that many patients diagnosed with AH report alcohol use over shorter periods of time before diagnosis. Heavy drinking has been defined as 15 or more drinks per week for men and 8 or more drinks per week for women.[2] In an Italian population study, the risk threshold for developing liver damage was ingestion of more than 30 g of alcohol per day in both men and women. The pattern of drinking was also an important determinant of hepatic damage; specifically, an increased risk was seen in patients drinking without food.[4] The type of alcohol use is also important; the risk of ALD was higher from drinking beer and spirits compared with drinking wine.[5]

In practice, most patients diagnosed with AH usually consume more than 100 g of alcohol per day, with higher consumption being associated with more severe disease. Binge drinking is defined by the National Institute on Alcohol Abuse and Alcoholism as the consumption of 5 or more drinks by a male or 4 or more drinks by a female in about 2 hours, resulting in a blood alcohol concentration of 0.08% or greater.[6] Despite limited quality data, binge drinking is a potential risk factor for AH, and is particularly thought to contribute to the rising incidence of AH in younger individuals. Importantly, a strong relationship between the prevalence of binge drinking and excessive drinking has been demonstrated in epidemiologic studies.[2] Although most patients diagnosed with AH are active drinkers, the disease can still be diagnosed after reducing or stopping alcohol consumption.

Risk Factors for Alcoholic Hepatitis

Aside from the quantity and pattern of alcohol consumption, a number of environmental and individual factors have been associated with the development of AH.

Age

AH is typically diagnosed in adults between with the ages of 40 and 50 years. However, as mentioned, younger patients are increasingly being diagnosed with AH, likely related to earlier heavy use of alcohol and binge drinking behavior.

Sex

Women are more prone to the toxic effects of alcohol and are at a greater risk of developing liver fibrosis and AH compared with men.[7,8] This gender susceptibility is attributed to several factors. Women have lower gastric levels of alcohol dehydrogenase, which lead to slower first-pass metabolism of alcohol. They have higher gut permeability leading to higher endotoxin levels after alcohol ingestion that promotes more oxidative stress and hepatic inflammation. Alcohol-mediated cytokine release from macrophages is greater in females. The greater body fat content in women also produces a lower volume of distribution for alcohol and therefore higher blood alcohol concentration after lesser volumes of alcohol ingestion.

Ethnicity
Hispanics are more likely to develop AH at a younger age compared with Caucasians, and both Hispanics and African Americans are more likely to develop ALD.[9,10] It is not clear whether this racial susceptibility is owing to genetic variations, different patterns of alcohol use/abuse, differences in socioeconomic status, and/or access to medical care.

Obesity
Obesity is an independent risk factor for cirrhosis in alcoholic patients and potentiates the severity of AH. The synergy between obesity and heavy alcohol intake likely is the result of similar disease mechanisms for both ALD and nonalcoholic fatty liver disease.[11]

Malnutrition
Protein–calorie malnutrition is a major risk factor for developing AH and is an indicator of poor outcomes and decreased survival in patients with established AH.[12]

Coexistent hepatitis C virus infection
The combination of alcohol use and hepatitis C virus infection has been associated with rapid progression to fibrosis and higher incidence of cirrhosis than either factor alone. In patients with AH, the presence of hepatitis C virus infection was demonstrated as an independent risk factor for higher mortality at 6 months.[13]

Hereditary factors
Monozygotic twins were shown to have a higher concordance rate for alcoholic cirrhosis than dizygotic twins.[14] Variations in the genes for cytochrome P450 2E1 (CYP2E1) and alcohol dehydrogenase; the major enzymes involved in alcohol metabolism, affect alcohol-driven tissue damage in addition to having a proposed influence on patterns of alcohol consumption and dependency, which in turn can predispose individuals to AH.[15]

CLINICAL PRESENTATION
Symptoms and Signs

The diagnosis of AH is primarily based on the clinical presentation (**Box 1**). Obtaining an accurate alcohol consumption history on presentation is crucial, although not always feasible. In symptomatic individuals, progressive jaundice is the main presenting feature, and a history of heavy alcohol use is typically elicited. Other clinical features can include fever, anorexia, weight loss, fatigue, generalized weakness, and nausea and vomiting. Patients can have complications related to portal hypertension such as ascites and variceal hemorrhage, even in the absence of underlying cirrhosis. Patients with AH are also prone to develop encephalopathy secondary to severe hepatic dysfunction. With most AH patients being active drinkers, they can exhibit severe forms of alcohol withdrawal after suddenly decreasing or discontinuing their alcohol use. Within the first 24 hours after the last drink, tachycardia, hypertension, irritability, and hyperreflexia can occur. Over the next few days, more dangerous

---

Box 1
Alcoholic hepatitis signs and symptoms

Nausea/vomiting

Abdominal pain (usually right upper quadrant and/or midepigastric)

Fatigue

Weakness

Anorexia

Jaundice

Fever

Increased abdominal girth with ascites

Hepatic encephalopathy

Variceal bleeding

Tender hepatomegaly

Hepatic bruit

Stigmata of chronic liver disease
  Spider angiomata
  Palmar erythema
  Gynecomastia
  Parotid enlargement
  Increased collateral vessels on anterior abdominal wall
  Dupuytren's contractures

---

complications including seizures and delirium tremens can arise. On physical examination tender hepatomegaly can be present, and occasionally a hepatic bruit can be auscultated, likely related to increased flow through the hepatic artery. Classical nonspecific signs of liver disease such as parotid enlargement, Dupuytren's contractures, dilated abdominal wall veins, and spider nevi can be present.[16]

Laboratory Findings

No single laboratory marker can definitively establish the diagnosis of AH, but a number of biochemical derangements can be seen in these patients. The classical finding is an elevated aspartate aminotransferase to 2 to 6 times the upper limit of normal (usually <300 IU/L) and elevation of alanine aminotransferase, to a lesser extent, resulting in an aspartate aminotransferase:alanine aminotransferase ratio of 2 or greater.[17] Leukocytosis with an elevated neutrophil count, anemia, and hyperbilirubinemia are common. Leukocytosis can be a feature of AH itself, as part of the systemic inflammatory response syndrome (SIRS), or an indication of underlying infection. In severe cases of AH, serum albumin can be low and coagulopathy with a prolonged prothrombin time (increased International Normalized Ratio) is common. Patients with AH are also prone to renal injury and approximately 7% can be diagnosed with hepatorenal syndrome type 1.[18]

Ruling out Infection

Patients with AH are especially prone to developing bacterial infections and about 25% of patients with severe AH have an infection at the time of presentation.[19] Indeed, infection is a leading cause of mortality in those with severe disease. Therefore, close monitoring for symptoms and signs of infection is crucial and screening for infections is warranted on admission as well as repeatedly during the hospital stay in patients who experience clinical deterioration. Routine blood and urine cultures should be obtained and paracentesis should be performed in those with ascites to evaluate for bacterial peritonitis. Importantly, patients with AH frequently have SIRS criteria that can be related to the overall inflammatory nature of the disease itself or can reflect an active bacterial infection. Regardless of the exact etiology, SIRS triggers a cascade of events that culminate in multiorgan failure, and an increased mortality risk is associated with increasing presence of the SIRS parameters.

Ruling out Other Liver Diseases

Other causes of acute liver injury such as drug-induced liver injury, viral hepatitis, autoimmune hepatitis, Wilsonian crisis, and cholangitis should be ruled out while evaluating patients with suspected AH. Liver, vascular, and biliary imaging are required to exclude biliary or vascular disorders as well as hepatocellular carcinoma.

DIAGNOSIS
Clinical Prognostic Scoring Models of Alcoholic Hepatitis

Based mainly on laboratory parameters, a number of scoring models are used to assess the severity of AH, predict mortality, and guide decisions for initiation of specific therapies.[20–23] For more information on scoring models please see Gholam PM: Prognosis and Prognostic Scoring Models for Alcoholic Liver Disease and Acute Alcoholic Hepatitis, in this issue. The Maddrey discriminant function remains widely used in the initial assessment of patients with AH. A value of 32 or greater signifies severe disease and has been used as a threshold for initiation of corticosteroid therapy in the absence of other contraindications.[20] The role of the Model for End-stage Liver Disease (MELD) score has been evaluated in assessing the severity of AH. A MELD score of 21 has been reported to have the highest sensitivity and specificity to predict mortality in patients with AH, estimating a 90-day mortality of 20% for patients with this score.[21] A MELD score of 21 has also been used as a threshold for starting corticosteroid therapy.[24] In addition to the role of the MELD score in the initial assessment of AH patients, a progressive increase in MELD score in hospitalized AH patients is associated with significantly poor outcomes and higher in-hospital mortality.[25] Although the Glasgow Alcoholic Hepatitis Score and the ABIC (age, serum bilirubin, International Normalized Ratio, and serum creatinine) scores have been shown to predict survival outcomes in patients with AH, their use has been limited owing to lack of external validation studies.[22,23] Finally, the Lille score was designed to assess the response of patients with severe AH to corticosteroid therapy. It is calculated based on 5 pretreatment variables (age, albumin, prothrombin time, bilirubin on day 0 of treatment, and presence or absence of renal insufficiency) and the change in bilirubin at day 7 of treatment. A Lille score of 0.45 or greater is associated with 75% mortality at 6 months, indicating that corticosteroids should be discontinued owing to lack of response.[26]

Role of Liver Biopsy

Although the diagnosis of AH is suspected based on clinical and biochemical data, a definitive diagnosis may require histologic confirmation and a liver biopsy remains the "gold standard" diagnostic tool. According the guidelines of American Association for the Study of Liver Diseases, a liver biopsy should be considered when contemplating medical treatment for patients with a clinical diagnosis of severe AH, and in patients without a clear underlying diagnosis.[27] Findings on liver biopsy in AH include steatosis, hepatocyte ballooning, neutrophil infiltration, Mallory bodies (aggregated cytokeratin intermediate filaments and other proteins), and scarring with a typical perivenular distribution compared with the periportal fibrosis observed in chronic viral hepatitis. Limitations of liver biopsy include cost, sampling errors, and interobserver variability. The percutaneous approach carries the risk of serious complications, such as bleeding, infection, pneumothorax, hemothorax, and organ puncture.[28] The usefulness of liver biopsy in patients with AH is particularly controversial, because many of these patients are coagulopathic and have thrombocytopenia and/or ascites, all of which can complicate or prevent a percutaneous liver biopsy. Therefore, a transjugular liver biopsy is preferred in this setting, but this procedure is not widely available outside tertiary medical centers.

Histologic Prognostic Scoring of Alcoholic Hepatitis

In addition to aiding in the diagnosis of AH, liver biopsy may have a role in determining AH prognosis. A recent multicenter study has tested and validated an Alcoholic Hepatitis Histologic Score (AHHS), and showed its accuracy in predicting short-term mortality in patients with AH.[29] This study included 121 patients with biopsy-proven AH as the initial set, with subsequent testing and updating of the score in a test set of 96 patients, then validation in an independent set of 109 patients. The AHHS was generated using 4 histologic features that independently predicted short-term survival: stage of fibrosis, degree of neutrophil infiltration, pattern of bilirubinostasis, and presence of mega mitochondria. Optimal cutoff values to define different severity categories were 3 and 6 points (sensitivity of 98%, 72% and specificity of 20%, 75%, respectively). Using these cutoff values, the AHHS identified patients with AH as having low (0–3 points), moderate (4–5 points), or high (6–9 points) 90-day mortality rates. None of the individual histologic features assessed by the AHHS were useful in predicting response to corticosteroid therapy. This study also demonstrated an association between the pattern of bilirubinostasis and the risk of developing a bacterial infection during hospitalization, because nearly 50% of patients with canalicular/ductular bilirubinostasis or hepatocellular plus canalicular/ductular bilirubinostasis developed a bacterial infection during hospitalization. The degree of bilirubinostasis itself progressed with increasing levels of serum bilirubin. **Table 1** summarizes the AHHS calculation.

Table 1 Alcoholic Hepatitis Histologic Score	
Component	**Points**
Stage of fibrosis	No fibrosis or portal fibrosis 0 Expansive fibrosis 0 Bridging fibrosis or cirrhosis +3
Degree of neutrophil infiltration	No or mild +2 Severe 0
Pattern of bilirubinostasis	No 0 Hepatocellular only 0 Canalicular/ductular +1 Hepatocellular plus canalicular/ductular +2
Mega mitochondria	No +2 Yes 0

Score is calculated by sum of all points.
   Alcoholic hepatitis severity: mild (0–3 points), intermediate (4–5 points), severe (6–9 points).
   Data from Altamirano J, Miquel R, Katoonizadeh A, et al. A histologic scoring system for prognosis of patients with alcoholic hepatitis. Gastroenterology 2014;146:1231–9.e1–6.

Noninvasive Diagnostic Modalities

Given the limitations and potential complications of liver biopsy, there is a need for alternative noninvasive methods for AH diagnosis and assessment of disease severity. Analysis of breath biomarkers, including volatile organic compounds and elemental gases, have been evaluated recently in the diagnosis of AH. A study reported a diagnostic model using the combination of the breath levels of trimethylamine and pentane to distinguish patients with AH from those with acute liver decompensation from causes other than alcohol or controls without liver disease.[30] This model, known as TAP, provided accurate prediction for the diagnosis of AH with 90% sensitivity and 80% specificity for a TAP score of 36 or higher. The levels of exhaled trimethylamine had a low level of correlation with the severity of AH based on MELD score. These results need to be validated externally.

OUTCOMES
Short-Term and Long-Term Survival

The natural history of AH is variable and depends on the severity of the disease, whether treatment is initiated or not, and abstinence from further alcohol use. In a pooled analysis of 19 clinical trials of AH, the overall mortality was about 34% among 661 patients randomized to placebo.[31] The 1-month mortality rate in trials that included patients with severe AH was approximately 23%. The leading cause of death in these patients was liver failure followed by gastrointestinal bleeding and infection. The high short-term mortality of severe AH was also demonstrated in a metaanalysis of 5 randomized controlled trials that evaluated the role of corticosteroid treatment.[32] The 28-day mortality rate in 197 non–corticosteroid-treated patients with severe AH was 34.3%. Short-term mortality in patients with mild to moderate AH is less well-reported, but is generally low.

Although the high short-term mortality associated with severe AH is well-reported, long-term survival after AH is not as well-described. A recent study demonstrated a significant correlation between the long-term survival after an episode of AH with abstinence from alcohol.[33] In this study, the estimated 5-year overall survival rate was 31.8%, with a 3-fold higher survival rate in abstainers compared with relapsed and continued drinkers. About one-half of patients surviving the index hospitalization died during the study follow-up period.

Progression to Cirrhosis

Many patients already have underlying alcoholic cirrhosis at the time of initial AH presentation. In those without cirrhosis, progression to cirrhosis primarily depends on continued consumption of alcohol, but an older study reported that about 10% to 20% of patients with AH progress to cirrhosis every year, with 70% of all patients ultimately developing cirrhosis.[34] Women diagnosed with AH are a higher risk of progression to cirrhosis than men despite abstinence.[35] Total abstinence from alcohol use can lead to complete return of normal liver histology in about 10% of patients with AH.

Recidivism

Abstinence from alcohol use is the cornerstone of management in patients with AH and complete sobriety is vital for recovery of liver injury. Data on the prevalence and patterns of recidivism after the diagnosis of AH is limited and its impact on patient survival is conflicting. Studies have reported a recidivism rate of 28% at 6 months and 37% at 12 months in patients with severe AH.[23,36] A more recent retrospective study from the United Kingdom analyzed data from 109 patients hospitalized for severe AH, with an aim of assessing their long-term outcomes, including survival and recidivism.[33] During a median follow-up of 40.7 months from hospitalization, 63 patients died (57.8%) including 22 who died during the index hospitalization. The other 41 patients had a median survival of 30.2 months. Among 87 patients surviving the index hospitalization, 57% were drinking at time of last follow-up, including two-thirds who continued to drink and one-third who relapsed after initial abstinence. Another 8% suffered an alcohol relapse but were eventual abstainers at time of last follow-up. Abstinence at last follow-up was the only independent predictor of long-term outcome, with the 5-year survival being approximately 3-fold higher in abstainers (75.3%) compared with relapsed drinkers (26.8%) and continued drinkers (21.0%; $P = .005$). Importantly, this study showed that the survival benefit from sobriety in AH was not apparent until 18 months after discharge (hazard ratio, 2.714; 95% CI, 0.995–7.404; $P = .051$), and that transient abstinence is of little benefit in AH patients indicating the need for immediate and sustained sobriety. Therefore, medical therapy to decrease alcohol relapse after recovery from AH should be considered to lower the high rate of recidivism. Interestingly, among 12 patients who underwent a liver biopsy in this study, 11 (91.7%) had underlying cirrhosis, and an additional 83 had evidence of cirrhosis based on imaging studies, for a total of 86.2%, consistent with prior reports of the high prevalence of cirrhosis in patients diagnosed with AH.[33]

Recurrent Alcoholic Hepatitis

Recurrence of AH has been reported to account for 2.4% to 18% of diagnosed AH episodes.[23,37] The recurrent episodes of AH followed short periods of recidivism with marked clinical and biochemical improvement during the intervening periods of abstinence. Recurrent episodes of AH have been reported to be more severe and protracted, as reflected by worse prognostic scores including discriminant function (70.4 ± 27.9 vs 50.5 ± 10.9; $P = .014$) and MELD score (26.2 ± 3.7 vs 22.1 ± 1.5; $P = .008$) as well as having a higher prevalence of complications.[37] When compared with other AH patients who had recidivism, those who developed recurrent AH had similar mortality (about 57%), but a greater number of hospital admissions than expected. These findings again indicate that recidivism itself is a significant predictor of poor outcomes in patients with AH.

REFERENCES

1. Rehm J, Samokhvalov AV, Shield KD. Global burden of alcoholic liver diseases. J Hepatol 2013;59(1):160–8.
2. Esser MB, Hedden SL, Kanny D, et al. Prevalence of alcohol dependence among US adult drinkers, 2009–2011. Prev Chronic Dis 2014;11:E206.
3. Liangpunsakul S. Clinical characteristics and mortality of hospitalized alcoholic hepatitis patients in the United States. J Clin Gastroenterol 2011;45(8):714–9.
4. Bellentani S, Saccoccio G, Costa G, et al. Drinking habits as cofactors of risk for alcohol induced liver damage. Gut 1997;41:845–50.
5. Becker U, Grønbaek M, Johansen D, et al. Lower risk for alcohol-induced cirrhosis in wine drinkers. Hepatology 2002;35(4):868–75.
6. Zakhari S, Li TK. Determinants of alcohol use and abuse: impact of quantity and frequency patterns on liver disease. Hepatology 2007;46:2032–9.
7. Sato N, Lindros KO, Baraona E, et al. Sex difference in alcohol-related organ injury. Alcohol Clin Exp Res 2001;25(5 Suppl ISBRA):40S–5S.

8. Bird GL, Williams R. Factors determining cirrhosis in alcoholic liver disease. Mol Aspects Med 1988;10:97–105.
9. Levy RE, Catana AM, Durbin-Johnson B, et al. Ethnic differences in presentation and severity of alcoholic liver disease. Alcohol Clin Exp Res 2015;39:566–74.
10. Caetano R, Kaskutas LA. Changes in drinking patterns among whites, blacks and Hispanics, 1984-1992. J Stud Alcohol 1995;56(5):558–65.
11. Naveau S, Giraud V, Borotto E, et al. Excess weight risk factor for alcoholic liver disease. Hepatology 1997;25:108–11.
12. Mendenhall C, Roselle GA, Gartside P, et al. The relationship of protein calorie malnutrition to alcoholic liver disease: a reexamination of data from two Veterans Administration Cooperative Studies. Alcohol Clin Exp Res 1995;19(6):635–41.
13. Singal AK, Sagi S, Kuo YF, et al. Impact of hepatitis C virus infection on the course and outcome of patients with acute alcoholic hepatitis. Eur J Gastroenterol Hepatol 2011;23(3):204–9.
14. Hrubec Z, Omenn GS. Evidence of genetic predisposition to alcoholic cirrhosis and psychosis: twin concordances for alcoholism and its biological end points by zygosity among male veterans. Alcohol Clin Exp Res 1981;5:207–15.
15. Seitz HK, Stickel F. Risk factors and mechanisms of hepatocarcinogenesis with special emphasis on alcohol and oxidative stress. Biol Chem 2006;387(4): 349–60.
16. Dugum M, Zein N, McCullough A, et al. Alcoholic hepatitis: challenges in diagnosis and management. Cleve Clin J Med 2015;82(4):226–36.
17. Cohen JA, Kaplan MM. The SGOT/SGPT ratio–an indicator of alcoholic liver disease. Dig Dis Sci 1979;24(11):835–8.
18. Lucey MR, Mathurin P, Morgan TR. Alcoholic hepatitis. N Engl J Med 2009;360(6): 2758–69.
19. Louvet A, Wartel F, Castel H, et al. Infection in patients with severe alcoholic hepatitis treated with steroids: early response to therapy is the key factor. Gastroenterology 2009;137(2):541–8.
20. Maddrey WC, Boitnott JK, Bedine MS, et al. Corticosteroid therapy of alcoholic hepatitis. Gastroenterology 1978;75(8):193–9.
21. Sheth M, Riggs M, Patel T. Utility of the Mayo End-Stage Liver Disease (MELD) score in assessing prognosis of patients with alcoholic hepatitis. BMC Gastroenterol 2002;2:2.
22. Forrest EH, Morris AJ, Stewart S, et al. The Glasgow alcoholic hepatitis score identifies patients who may benefit from corticosteroids. Gut 2007;56(12):1743–6.
23. Dominguez M, Rincon D, Abraldes JG, et al. A new scoring system for prognostic stratification of patients with alcoholic hepatitis. Am J Gastroenterol 2008;103(11): 2747–56.
24. Dunn W, Jamil LH, Brown LS, et al. MELD accurately predicts mortality in patients with alcoholic hepatitis. Hepatology 2005;41(2):353–8.
25. Srikureja W, Kyulo NL, Runyon BA, et al. MELD score is a better prognostic model than Child-Turcotte-Pugh score or discriminant function score in patients with alcoholic hepatitis. J Hepatol 2005;42(5):700–6.
26. Louvet A, Naveau S, Abdelnour M, et al. The Lille model: a new tool for therapeutic strategy in patients with severe alcoholic hepatitis treated with steroids. Hepatology 2007;45(6):1348–54.
27. O'Shea RS, Dasarathy S, McCullough AJ, Practice Guideline Committee of the American Association for the Study of Liver Diseases, Practice Parameters Committee of the American College of Gastroenterology. Alcoholic liver disease. Hepatology 2010;51(1):307–28.

28. Bravo AA, Sheth SG, Chopra S. Liver biopsy. N Engl J Med 2001;344(2):495–500.
29. Altamirano J, Miquel R, Katoonizadeh A, et al. A histologic scoring system for prognosis of patients with alcoholic hepatitis. Gastroenterology 2014;146: 1231–9.e1-6.
30. Hanouneh IA, Zein NN, Cikach F, et al. The breathprints in patients with liver disease identify novel breath biomarkers in alcoholic hepatitis. Clin Gastroenterol Hepatol 2014;12(3):516–23.
31. Yu CH, Xu CF, Ye H, et al. Early mortality of alcoholic hepatitis: a review of data from placebo controlled clinical trials. World J Gastroenterol 2010;16(5):2435–9.
32. Mathurin P, O'Grady J, Carithers RL, et al. Corticosteroids improve short-term survival in patients with severe alcoholic hepatitis: meta-analysis of individual patient data. Gut 2011;60(2):255–60.
33. Potts JR, Goubet S, Heneghan MA, et al. Determinants of long-term outcome in severe alcoholic hepatitis. Aliment Pharmacol Ther 2013;38:584–95.
34. Pares A, Caballeria J, Bruguera M, et al. Histological course of alcoholic hepatitis. Influence of abstinence, sex and extent of hepatic damage. J Hepatol 1986;2: 33–42.
35. Raynard B, Balian A, Fallik D, et al. Risk factors of fibrosis in alcohol-induced liver disease. Hepatology 2002;35(3):635–8.
36. Mathurin P, Abdelnour M, Ramond MJ, et al. Early change in bilirubin levels is an important prognostic factor in severe alcoholic hepatitis treated with prednisolone. Hepatology 2003;38:1363–9.
37. Potts JR, Howard MR, Verma S. Recurrent severe alcoholic hepatitis: clinical characteristics and outcomes. Eur J Gastroenterol Hepatol 2013;25:659–64.

Acute Alcoholic Hepatitis: Therapy

Paulina K. Phillips, MD, Michael R. Lucey, MD*

KEYWORDS

- Corticosteroids • Prednisolone • Pentoxifylline • Nutrition • Anti-TNFα
- Antioxidants • Liver transplantation • Palliative care

KEY POINTS

- Alcoholic hepatitis (AH) carries significant morbidity and mortality.
- Every patient with AH should be advised to stop all alcohol consumption and should be provided with sufficient nutrition.
- Those patients who meet the criteria for severe AH should be considered for therapy with prednisolone, and all patients with severe AH who fail medical therapy should be considered for liver transplantation (LT).
- All patients with severe AH who fail medical therapy and are considered unsuitable for LT should be referred for palliative care consultation.

INTRODUCTION

Alcoholic hepatitis (AH) is a term used to describe both a clinical syndrome and a set of histopathologic findings. AH occurs in the setting of alcohol use disorder (in common parlance, *alcoholism*). All treatment of AH begins with the premise that patients need to establish and maintain abstinence from alcohol. Assessment of the psychological state is an important element in the holistic care of an individual patient with severe AH, but this is beyond the scope of the article. Similarly, because many patients with AH have been drinking up to the moment of admission to the hospital, care of patients at risk for alcohol withdrawal syndrome is key to the recovery process. Management of alcohol withdrawal syndrome has been thoroughly reviewed elsewhere and is not covered here.[1] Finally, it is worth stating that severe AH usually arises in patients with established cirrhosis, although patients are often unaware of this fact. Consequently, as mentioned in the *Patient evaluation overview* section, typical patients with AH are at risk for the other end-organ failures seen in sick cirrhotic patients.

The authors have nothing to disclose.
Division of Gastroenterology and Hepatology, Department of Medicine, University of Wisconsin School of Medicine and Public Health, 1685 Highland Avenue, Madison, WI 53705-2281, USA
* Corresponding author.
E-mail address: mrl@medicine.wisc.edu

Clin Liver Dis 20 (2016) 509–519
http://dx.doi.org/10.1016/j.cld.2016.02.015

Box 1

Five controversies regarding the evaluation and treatment of alcoholic hepatitis

1. How to distinguish acute-on-chronic liver failure from AH

2. Need for liver biopsy to diagnose AH

3. Use of corticosteroids to treat severe AH

4. Role (if any) of liver transplantation to treat patients with ALD with short duration of sobriety

5. Role of palliative care in the management of patients with AH

Moreover, management of ascites; fluid and electrolyte imbalances; cardiovascular, respiratory, and renal function; and hepatic encephalopathy are alluded to only tangentially. The focus of this article is the current state of management of the AH syndrome itself. In particular, the authors address 5 controversies related to the evaluation and treatment of patients with AH as shown in **Box 1.**

PATIENT EVALUATION OVERVIEW

Evaluation of patients with a putative diagnosis of AH begins with a careful history, including questions about the most recent use of alcohol. The National Institute on Alcohol Abuse and Alcoholism's quantity and frequency questions are useful to gauge the amount of alcohol that patients have been consuming (**Box 2**). Taking a history of exposure to other drugs of addiction is essential. Next, it is wise to corroborate the addiction history with a close family member or friend.

For more information on diagnosis of alcoholic liver disease, please see Ryan E. Childers and Joseph Ahn: Diagnosis of Alcoholic Liver Disease: Key Foundations and New Developments, in this issue. We wish to draw attention to the importance of distinguishing between AH and 'acute on chronic liver failure' (ACLF). As mentioned earlier, most patients with severe AH have already progressed to cirrhosis of the liver, even though many are unaware of this fact. Therefore, many are vulnerable to infection (**Box 3**). AH is a form of systemic inflammatory response syndrome (SIRS) that shares many features with systemic infection (**Box 4**). Common causes of infection in patients with ALD include pneumonia, spontaneous bacterial peritonitis in patients with ascites, urinary tract infection, cellulitis, and *Clostridium difficile* enterocolitis.[2] Hospitalized patients are prone to intravenous (IV) catheter–associated or urinary catheter–associated infections. Failure to recognize infection and/or difficulty distinguishing between AH and SIRS-like conditions that mimic AH confound day-to-day clinical practice and potentially contaminate the study populations in clinical trials. Chronic exposure to proton pump inhibitors and antibiotics also increase the infection risk in cirrhotic patients.

Box 2

National Institute on Alcohol Abuse and Alcoholism's quantity and frequency questions

1. On average, how many days per week do you drink alcohol?

2. On a typical day when you drink, how many drinks do you have?

3. What is the maximum number of drinks you had on any given occasion during the last month?

Box 3
Risk factors for infection in patients with alcoholic cirrhosis

- Immunocompromised by malnutrition and impaired liver function
- Aspiration after vomiting or upper endoscopy
- Low albumin ascites; risk for spontaneous bacterial peritonitis
- Urinary catheters: risk for urinary tract infection (CAUTI)
- Chronic use of antibiotics and PPIs increasing risk of infection (especially due to *Clostridium difficile*)

Abbreviations: CAUTI, catheter-associated urinary tract infection; PPIs, proton pump inhibitors.

Liver biopsy offers the best method to confirm the presence of AH and also to identify patients without the histopathologic features of AH despite a clinical syndrome that mimics it. However, there is a distinct variance in clinical practice regarding the role of liver biopsy in the diagnosis of AH between France and Spain, where liver biopsies are the norm, and the United States and United Kingdom, where they are infrequent. This difference in practice has potential significance in the studies of therapy for severe AH from the different countries, as is discussed later. In both clinical practice and clinical trials, the authors advocate the use of transjugular liver biopsy whenever there is reasonable doubt regarding the accuracy of the diagnosis of AH as a cause of severe liver injury.

The decision to admit patients with putative AH to the hospital and to initiate pharmacotherapy is greatly influenced by the clinician's assessment of patients' prognosis. For more information on prognostic scoring models, please see Pierre M. Gholam: Prognosis and Prognostic Scoring Models for Alcoholic Liver Disease and Acute Alcoholic Hepatitis, in this issue. Milder forms of AH have an excellent prognosis with clinical management of complications and cessation of alcohol, without the need to consider specific agents to counter the effects of AH. On the other hand, the short-term mortality can be high in patients with a Maddrey discriminant function (MDF) of 32 or greater. These patients are those in whom pharmacologic intervention, in addition to abstinence from alcohol, may have a salutary effect. Furthermore, the observation by Mathurin and colleagues[3] that an early decline in serum bilirubin when treated with prednisolone was a good prognostic sign led to the development of the Lille score. This score is calculated on day 7 of prednisolone therapy for severe AH and gives an indication as to whether patients are showing signs of recovery, in which case continuing corticosteroid for a full 28-day course makes good clinical sense, whereas failure to improve during the first 7 days allows the managing team to stop prednisolone before it causes harm to patients. Furthermore, Altamirano and colleagues[4] have recently reported on the prognostic (as opposed to diagnostic) value of liver biopsy.

Box 4
Features of systemic inflammatory response syndrome common to alcoholic hepatitis and acute-on-chronic liver failure

- Leukocytosis
- Tachycardia
- Systemic hypotension

TREATMENT OF ALCOHOLIC HEPATITIS: OVERVIEW

As stated earlier, abstinence from alcohol is the *sine qua non* of treating any form of ALD, including AH. As shown in **Fig. 1**, among a cohort of patients with biopsy-documented AH, survival was much worse in those patients who continued to drink heavily compared with those who reduced or stopped drinking.[5] Indeed, the capacity of the injured liver to resolve with (relatively) simple medical management confounds the study of both pharmacologic treatments and transplant surgery. In fact, one of the caveats expressed about the adoption of liver transplantation to treat patients with AH that has been unresponsive to medical management is that up to 25% of these patients would have recovered nonetheless, had the medical course been extended.[6]

The treatment of alcohol use disorder has never been studied at the time of presentation with AH, and no data-based account is possible with regards to either 'talking therapies' or pharmacotherapies. Therefore, the authors are left to describe the approach used at their center. The authors encourage patients with a new diagnosis of AH to make a commitment to enroll in formal alcohol addiction counseling and treatment, once they have recovered sufficiently to participate. Because there are no studies of pharmacologic approaches to reduce cravings for alcohol or prevent continued drinking (ie, ameliorating reinforcement) in patients with AH, the authors eschew these agents, while they await well-conducted clinical trials of these interventions.

Patients with AH are frequently malnourished, and the degree of malnutrition correlates with severity of liver injury and outcome.[7] Nutritional assessment and support is, thus, an imperative aspect of therapy for AH (as with many forms of ALD). Unfortunately, evidence for a survival benefit of a specific nutritional supplementation regimen in managing AH is less convincing. In 2000, Cabré and colleagues[8] published an

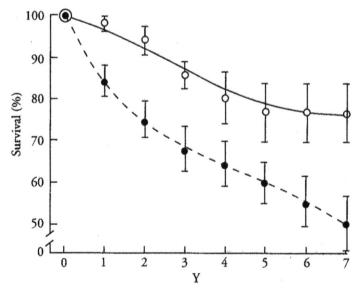

Fig. 1. Survival in 59 patients with biopsy-proven acute AH according to continued heavy (*closed circles*) or reduced (*open circles*) alcohol use. (*Data from* Lischner MW, Alexander JF, Galambos JT. Natural history of alcoholic hepatitis. I. The acute disease. Am J Dig Dis 1971;16:481–94.)

interim analysis of a prospective, multicenter, randomized controlled trial (RCT) comparing total enteral nutrition (2000 kcal/d) with prednisolone (40 mg/d) for 28 days in patients with severe AH. Unfortunately, the study is difficult to interpret, in part because it was underpowered and also because no final report with greater recruitment has since been published. Furthermore, the results are equivocal in that corticosteroids seemed to delay death during treatment when compared with supplemental enteral nutrition, whereas corticosteroids were followed by more deaths after the treatment period was complete. Recently, 2 meta-analyses examined the effects of nutritional supplementation in ALD, including AH, and neither found a survival benefit with nutritional supplements.[9,10] Based on the available data, the American Association for the Study of Liver Diseases' (AASLD) guideline is confined to a very general statement:

"All patients with alcoholic hepatitis or advanced ALD should be assessed for nutritional deficiencies (protein-calorie malnutrition), as well as vitamin and mineral deficiencies. Those with severe disease should be treated aggressively with enteral nutritional therapy (Class I, level B)."[11]

Because AH often arises in the setting of cirrhosis, all aspects of managing decompensated cirrhosis need to be considered, including salt restriction and judicious use of diuretics in the treatment of ascites, lactulose and rifaximin to combat hepatic encephalopathy, administration of albumin and vasoconstrictors in hepatorenal syndrome, antimicrobials for treatment of infection (when present), and supportive management of alcohol withdrawal.

PHARMACOLOGIC TREATMENT OPTIONS
Corticosteroids

Prednisone and its active metabolite, prednisolone, interact with the inflammatory response in several ways. These interactions include the inhibition of transcription factors, thereby decreasing circulating levels of proinflammatory cytokines interleukin 8 (IL-8) and tumor necrosis factor α (TNF-α), and a decrease in the expression of intracellular adhesion molecule 1. High-dose corticosteroids have become a cornerstone of therapy for severe AH. Prednisolone should not be started within 48 hours of a variceal hemorrhage or when uncontrolled infection is present. Once infection is being treated with appropriate antibiotics, prednisone can be started.[12]

Although the practice guidelines from both the AASLD and the European Association for the Study of the Liver recommend prednisolone 40 mg/d for 28 days (followed by discontinuation or a 2- to 4-week taper) in the treatment of severe AH, the use of corticosteroids to treat severe AH remains controversial.[11,13] The best evidence favoring their use comes from the 2011 meta-analysis by Mathurin and colleagues[14] of 5 RCTs totaling more than 400 patients, which demonstrated a significant 28-day survival benefit in patients with severe AH of 79.97 $\pm$ 2.8% in the treated subjects compared with 65.7 $\pm$ 3.4% ($P = .0005$) in the control subjects. Mathurin and colleagues introduced the Lille score as an instrument to determine on day 7 of treatment whether or not to continue therapy. As discussed earlier, the patients included in these studies were extremely ill, with a 28-day mortality of 34%.

However, there is a considerable body of literature that would argue against prednisolone as an effective therapy in severe AH. For example, a 2008 Cochrane meta-analysis of 15 trials (more than 700 patients) by Rambaldi and colleagues[15] showed no statistically significant reduction in mortality in the corticosteroid group compared with placebo or no intervention. Unfortunately, most of the trials were at high risk of bias owing to significant heterogeneity.

Recently, Thursz and colleagues[16] published a multicenter, double-blind, factorial (2 × 2) trial (the STOPAH [Steroids or Pentoxifylline for Alcoholic Hepatitis] trial) that randomized 1103 patients with AH with a DF of 32 or greater into one of 4 arms: placebo/placebo (ie, the natural history of the disease), prednisolone/placebo, pentoxifylline (PTX)/placebo, or prednisolone/PTX. All diagnoses were made on clinical criteria, and liver biopsies were not required. The power analysis was based on a predicted reduction in 28-day mortality from 30% (in the placebo/placebo group) to 21% (in the treated groups). In fact, the 28-day mortality in the placebo/placebo group was 17%, compared with 14% in the prednisolone/placebo group, 19% in the PTX/placebo group, and 13% in the prednisolone/PTX group. There was a nonsignificant survival advantage during the first 4 weeks among patients who received prednisolone (odds ratio [OR] 0.72; 95% confidence interval [CI] 0.52–1.01, $P = .06$). On cross-sectional analysis of 28-day survival, neither prednisolone nor PTX was associated with a survival benefit. However, on multivariable analysis, prednisolone was associated with improved 28-day survival, with an OR of survival of 0.609 ($P = .015$). The STOPAH trial has raised several important questions: Did the absence of liver biopsy distort the composition of the study groups? In particular, were some of the patients who were classified as having AH really cirrhotic patients with sepsis, representing acute-on-chronic liver disease rather than just pure AH. Alternatively, has the management of severe AH improved so that the 28-survival represented in STOPAH represents the new norm? These questions are prompted by the finding that the 28-day mortality in the pure control group was approximately half that reported in previous trials.

In summary, the Cochrane and STOPAH studies have dampened the enthusiasm for corticosteroids as a treatment of AH. In the authors' opinion, we continue to think that corticosteroids are useful for selected patients with severe AH in whom active infection is absent, with the caveat that they stop at day 7 in the absence of a favorable response, as judged by the Lille score.

Pentoxifylline

PTX, a nonselective phosphodiesterase inhibitor, modulates TNF-α transcription and reduces the formation of IL-5, IL-10, and IL-12. Its side effect profile ranges from gastrointestinal upset (nausea, vomiting, dyspepsia) to more serious, but also more rare, complications, including arrhythmias, hypotension, bleeding, and aseptic meningitis.[17]

The salutary effect of PTX in treating AH was promoted by the RCT of Akriviadis and colleagues,[18] in which 101 patients with severe AH were randomized to receive either PTX or placebo. The short-term mortality was 24.5% in the PTX group and 46.0% in the control group ($P = .04$). Serial TNF-α levels were monitored and did not differ significantly between both groups. Twenty-two of 24 deaths in the placebo arm were related to the hepatorenal syndrome (HRS), as compared with 6 of 12 in the PTX group ($P = .009$). Hence, the main benefit of PTX seemed to be the prevention of HRS in a vulnerable population. Criticisms of the study were that the investigators used a convenience rather than fixed observation period and that the entry criteria were arbitrary, with potential subjects excluded who were thought by the principal investigator to be improving or dying.

A 2009 Cochrane review of 5 RCTs (336 patients) comparing PTX with control showed a reduced mortality in the PTX arm (relative risk [RR] 0.64; 95% CI 0.46–0.89), but this was not supported by trial sequential analysis.[19] Further, owing to a high risk of bias in 4 of the 5 studies, there was concern that the intervention effect was overestimated. In a subsequent RCT, Mathurin and colleagues[20] failed to find an additional benefit of combining PTX with prednisolone, compared with prednisolone as a single agent. Also, PTX does not seem to be an effective rescue agent when substituted at day 7 in patients who are failing prednisone therapy.[21] Most recently, the STOPAH study failed to show any survival benefit for the use of pentoxifylline either alone or in combination with corticosteroids.

The AASLD's guideline currently supports the use of PTX, dosed at 400 mg orally 3 times per day for 28 days, in patients with severe AH with early renal failure or in those with a contraindication to corticosteroids (level B evidence).[11] Based on the accumulated studies cited earlier, we predict that this recommendation will be changed in the next iteration of the guideline to 'insufficient evidence to support the use of PTX in severe AH.'

Anti–Tumor Necrosis Factor α Agents

The commonly proposed pathophysiology of AH asserts that TNF-α produced by Kupffer cells interacts with TNF receptor 1, leading to the activation of caspases, mitochondrial injury, and eventual apoptosis of the hepatocyte.[22] Unfortunately, 2 well-constructed RCTs of biological agents (infliximab, etanercept) have failed to show a benefit.[23,24] Moreover, the side effect profile related to infection was unacceptable in each study. Based on all of the available data, anti-TNF-α agents are not recommended as therapy for AH outside of clinical trials.

Antioxidants

Reactive oxidant species may serve as mediators of alcohol-induced liver injury.[22,25] Consequently, several antioxidants have been studied, in combination with abstinence from alcohol, as treatments for AH. These agents include N-acetylcysteine (NAC), S-adenosyl-L-methionine (SAMe), and combinations of antioxidants, such as beta carotene, vitamin A, vitamin C, vitamin E, and selenium. In a study of 174 patients with severe AH randomized to receive either prednisolone alone or to prednisolone plus NAC, combination therapy decreased mortality significantly at 1 month (8% vs 24%, $P = .006$) but not at 3 months (22% vs 34%, $P = .06$) or 6 months (27% vs 38%, $P = .07$).[26] This study is well designed, which unfortunately had 6-month survival as its primary end point. Thus, although it did not meet its primary end point (improvement in 6-month survival), it suggests that NAC may have value in the treatment of severe AH. In another study, corticosteroids (oral prednisolone or IV methylprednisolone) were superior to an antioxidant cocktail in the treatment of severe AH, with 30-day mortality in the steroid group being 30% compared with 46% in the antioxidant group ($P = .05$).[27] Stewart and colleagues[28] further found that 6-month survival in severe AH was not improved in patients given antioxidant therapy, whether alone or in combination with corticosteroids.

Compared with placebo, vitamin E, which protects cell membranes against lipid peroxidation, has not been shown to improve survival in patients with severe AH.[29] SAMe is a methyl donor involved in glutathione synthesis. In 2006, a Cochrane report determined that there was insufficient evidence to either support or discourage the use of SAMe in ALD.[30] Similarly, Bjelakovic and colleagues[9] found, in a Cochrane review of 20 randomized trials involving various forms of ALD, including AH, that antioxidant supplements (beta carotene, vitamin A, vitamin C, vitamin E, and selenium) had no significant effect on all-cause mortality (RR 0.84, 95% CI 0.60–1.19, $I^2 = 0\%$) or liver-related mortality (RR 0.89, 95% CI 0.39–2.05, $I^2 = 37\%$). The AASLD's guidelines offer no direction on the use of antioxidants, which remain experimental agents at present.[11]

Miscellaneous Agents

Finally, there are tentative or preliminary data using many other agents in patients with severe AH. Calcium channel blockers (CCBs) have been found to have a hepatoprotective effect in animal models of alcohol-induced liver damage. However, in a small RCT, the dihydropyridine CCB amlodipine was not superior to placebo in improving survival in acute AH.[31] In view of the hypothetical importance of dysregulation of the balance between the gut microbiome and the intestinal mucosal barrier as a source of chronic inflammation in development of AH, modification of the gut microbiota and lipopolysaccharide pathway is an attractive therapeutic option. Studies manipulating the gut microbiome/gut mucosal barrier homeostasis have not (yet) been reported in patients with AH, although a pilot study of 66 adult Russian men admitted to a psychiatric hospital with a diagnosis of alcoholic psychosis randomized to receive a probiotic preparation (*Bifidobacterium bifidum* and *Lactobacillus plantarum 8PA3*) or standard therapy (abstinence and vitamins) suggested that probiotic supplementation led to improved serum aminotransferases.[32] Future studies will need to be performed before specific recommendations can be made in light of our relative ignorance of the complexity of gut microbiome/gut mucosal barrier homeostasis in the initiation and maintenance of ALD.[33]

In a pilot open-label study, 23 subjects with severe AH received granulocyte colony-stimulating factor, compared with 23 subjects receiving standard therapy; the treatment group showed a significant reduction in Model for End-Stage Liver Disease (MELD), MDF, and Child-Turcotte-Pugh scores at 1, 2, and 3 months.[34] Survival in the intervention group was also substantially increased at 90 days (78.3% vs 30.4%, $P = .001$). Finally, 30-day survival in patients with moderate or severe AH randomized to receive the anabolic steroid oxandrolone was not improved compared with the placebo group.[35]

SURGICAL TREATMENT OPTIONS
Liver Transplantation

For more information on the role of liver transplantation (LT) as a treatment of last resort in patients with ALD, please see Juan F. Gallegos-Orozco and Michael R. Charlton: Alcoholic liver disease and liver transplantation, in this issue. Severe AH that has failed medical management presents special challenges in this regard. In a landmark study, Mathurin and colleagues[36] demonstrated a mortality benefit in 26 patients with severe AH who had failed to respond to prednisolone for 7 days. All of the patients were experiencing their first episode of AH and had a median Lille score of 0.880 (range 0.260–0.996) and MELD score of 28.5 (range 23.0–52.4), indicating severe disease refractory to medical therapy and a high risk of mortality. Additional listing criteria included a good support group, commitment to abstinence from alcohol, and lack of severe coexisting conditions. Six-month survival was $77 \pm 8\%$ in transplant recipients, compared with $23 \pm 8\%$ in the matched historical cohort that did not receive a transplant ($P<.001$). This benefit was also significant at 24 months ($71 \pm 9\%$ survival in the transplant group vs $23 \pm 8\%$ in the nontransplant group, $P<.001$). Alcoholic relapse occurred in 3 patients (12%): one at 720 days, one at 740 days, and one at 1140 days after transplantation. Since then, Im and colleagues[37] have replicated these findings in a single-center study in the United States, once again showing excellent short-term survival in a group of patients with AH with a high risk of mortality.

Although LT can be seen as a life-saving procedure for some patients with severe AH, there is no consensus in the United States on how to identify these patients, on the appropriate selection criteria and the converse criteria to deny LT, or on the relative roles of the various voices in the discussion: physicians in the LT programs and other professionals, such as medical social workers, nurses, addiction counselors, patient representatives, administrators, and third-party payers. Also, it is unclear whether the general public would embrace LT for this particular indication (who ultimately donate the necessary organs). For patients with life-threatening AH who are denied LT, some may ultimately recover with medical management, although many will not. For these individuals, palliative care services are helpful for patients, the patients' families, and the medical team.[38,39]

SUMMARY

AH carries significant morbidity and mortality. Every patient with AH should be advised to stop all alcohol consumption and should be provided with sufficient nutrition. Those patients who meet the criteria for severe AH should be considered for therapy with prednisolone, and all patients with severe AH who fail medical therapy should be considered for LT. All patients with severe AH who fail medical therapy and are considered unsuitable for LT should be referred for palliative care consultation.

REFERENCES

1. Schuckit MA. Recognition and management of withdrawal delirium (delirium tremens). N Engl J Med 2014;371:2109–13.
2. O'Leary JG, Reddy KR, Wong F, et al. Long-term use of antibiotics and proton pump inhibitors predict development of infections in patients with cirrhosis. Clin Gastroenterol Hepatol 2015;13:753–9.e1–2.
3. Louvet A, Naveau S, Abdelnour M, et al. The Lille model: a new tool for therapeutic strategy in patients with severe alcoholic hepatitis treated with steroids. Hepatology 2007;45:1348–54.
4. Altamirano J, Miquel R, Katoonizadeh A, et al. A histologic scoring system for prognosis of patients with alcoholic hepatitis. Gastroenterology 2014;146:1231–9.
5. Lischner MW, Alexander JF, Galambos JT. Natural history of alcoholic hepatitis. I. The acute disease. Am J Dig Dis 1971;16:481–94.
6. Forrest EH, Lucey MR. Rescue liver transplantation for severe alcoholic hepatitis: arriving where we started? Hepatology 2013;57(1):10–2.
7. Mendenhall CL, Anderson S, Weesner RE, et al. Protein-calorie malnutrition associated with alcoholic hepatitis. Veterans Administration Cooperative Study Group on Alcoholic Hepatitis. Am J Med 1984;76:211–22.
8. Cabré E, Rodriguez-Iglesias P, Caballeria J, et al. Short- and long-term outcome of severe alcohol-induced hepatitis treated with steroids or enteral nutrition: a multicenter randomized trial. Hepatology 2000;32:36–42.
9. Bjelakovic G, Gluud LL, Nikolova D, et al. Antioxidant supplements for liver diseases. Cochrane Database Syst Rev 2011;(3):CD007749.
10. Koretz RL, Avenell A, Lipman TO. Nutritional support for liver disease. Cochrane Database Syst Rev 2012;(5):CD008344.
11. O'Shea RS, Dasarathy S, McCullough AJ. Alcoholic liver disease. Hepatology 2010;51(1):315–22.
12. Louvet A, Wartel F, Castel H, et al. Infection in patients with severe alcoholic hepatitis treated with steroids: early response to therapy is the key factor. Gastroenterology 2009;137:541–8.
13. Mathurin P, Hadengue A, Bataller R, et al. EASL clinical practical guidelines: management of alcoholic liver disease. J Hepatol 2012;57:399–420.
14. Mathurin P, O'Grady J, Carithers RL, et al. Corticosteroids improve short-term survival in patients with severe alcoholic hepatitis: meta-analysis of individual patient data. Gut 2011;60:255–60.

15. Rambaldi A, Saconato HH, Christensen E, et al. Systematic review: glucocorticosteroids for alcoholic hepatitis - a Cochrane Hepato-Biliary Group systematic review with meta-analyses and trial sequential analyses of randomized clinical trials. Aliment Pharmacol Ther 2008;27:1167–78.
16. Thursz MR, Richardson R, Allison M, et al. Prednisolone or pentoxifylline for alcoholic hepatitis. N Engl J Med 2015;372:1619–28.
17. Product information: TRENTAL(R) oral tablets, pentoxifylline oral tablets. Bridgewater (NJ): Sanofi-Aventis U.S. LLC (per FDA); 2012. Cited by 'Micromedix@. Available at: http://www.micromedexsolutions.com/micromedex2/librarian/PFDefaultActionId/evidencexpert.DoIntegratedSearch#close. Accessed November 1, 2015.
18. Akriviadis E, Botla R, Briggs W, et al. Pentoxifylline improves short-term survival in severe acute alcoholic hepatitis: a double-blind, placebo-controlled trial. Gastroenterology 2000;119:1637–48.
19. Whitfield K, Rambaldi A, Wetterslev J, et al. Pentoxifylline for alcoholic hepatitis. Cochrane Database Syst Rev 2009;(4):CD007339.
20. Mathurin P, Louvet A, Duhamel A, et al. Prednisolone with vs without pentoxifylline and survival of patients with severe alcoholic hepatitis: a randomized clinical trial. JAMA 2013;310(10):1033–41.
21. Louvet A, Diaz E, Dharancy S, et al. Early switch to pentoxifylline in patients with severe alcoholic hepatitis is inefficient in non-responders to corticosteroids. J Hepatol 2008;48:465–70.
22. Lucey MR, Mathurin P, Morgan TR. Alcoholic hepatitis. N Engl J Med 2009;360:2758–69.
23. Boetticher NC, Peine CJ, Kwo P, et al. A randomized, double-blinded, placebo-controlled multicenter trial of etanercept in the treatment of alcoholic hepatitis. Gastroenterology 2008;135:1953–60.
24. Naveau S, Chollet-Martin S, Dharancy S, et al. A double-blind randomized controlled trial of infliximab associated with prednisolone in acute alcoholic hepatitis. Hepatology 2004;39(5):1390–7.
25. Meagher EA, Barry OP, Burke A, et al. Alcohol-induced generation of lipid peroxidation products in humans. J Clin Invest 1999;104:805–13.
26. Nguyen-Khac E, Thevenot T, Piquet MA, et al. Glucocorticoids plus n-acetylcysteine in severe alcoholic hepatitis. N Engl J Med 2011;365:1781–9.
27. Phillips M, Curtis H, Portmann B, et al. Antioxidants versus corticosteroids in the treatment of severe alcoholic hepatitis-a randomised clinical trial. J Hepatol 2006;44:784–90.
28. Stewart S, Prince M, Bassendine M, et al. A randomized trial of antioxidant therapy alone or with corticosteroids in acute alcoholic hepatitis. J Hepatol 2007;47:277–83.
29. Mezey E, Potter JJ, Rennie-Tankersley L, et al. A randomized placebo controlled trial of vitamin E for alcoholic hepatitis. J Hepatol 2004;40:40–6.
30. Rambaldi A, Gluud C. S-adenosyl-L-methionine for alcoholic liver diseases (Review). Cochrane Database Syst Rev 2006;(2):CD002235.
31. Bird GL, Prach AT, McMahon AD, et al. Randomised controlled double-blind trial of the calcium channel antagonist amlodipine in the treatment of acute alcoholic hepatitis. J Hepatol 1998;28:194–8.
32. Kirpich IA, Solovieva NV, Leikhter SN, et al. Probiotics restore bowel flora and improve liver enzymes in human alcohol-induced liver injury: a pilot study. Alcohol 2008;42(8):675–82.
33. Kirpich IA, Parajuli D, McClain CJ. The gut microbiome in NAFLD and ALD. Clin Liver Dis 2015;6:55–8.

34. Singh V, Sharma AK, Narasimhan RL, et al. Granulocyte colony-stimulating factor in severe alcoholic hepatitis: a randomized pilot study. Am J Gastroenterol 2014; 109:1417–23.
35. Mendenhall CL, Anderson S, Garcia-Pont P, et al. Short-term and long-term survival in patients with alcoholic hepatitis treated with oxandrolone and prednisolone. N Engl J Med 1984;311:1464–70.
36. Mathurin P, Moreno C, Samuel D, et al. Early liver transplantation for severe alcoholic hepatitis. N Engl J Med 2011;365:1790–800.
37. Im G, Kim-Schluger L, Shenoy A, et al. Early liver transplantation for severe alcoholic hepatitis in the United States - a single center experience. Am J Transplant 2016;16(3):841–9.
38. Rakoski MO, Volk ML. Palliative care for patients with end-stage liver disease: an overview. Clin Liver Dis 2015;6:19–21.
39. Boyd K, Kimbell B, Murray S, et al. A "good death" with irreversible liver disease: talking with patients and families about deteriorating health and dying. Clin Liver Dis 2015;6:15–8.

Alcoholic Liver Disease and Liver Transplantation

Juan F. Gallegos-Orozco, MD[a], Michael R. Charlton, MD, FRCP[b],*

KEYWORDS

- Liver transplant • Alcohol use disorder • Alcoholic liver disease • Recidivism

KEY POINTS

- Excessive alcohol use is a common health care problem worldwide and is associated with significant morbidity and mortality.
- Alcoholic liver disease represents the second most frequent indication for liver transplantation in North America and Europe.
- The pretransplant evaluation of patients with alcoholic liver disease should aim at identifying those at high risk for posttransplant relapse of alcohol use disorder, as return to excessive drinking can be deleterious to graft and patient survival.
- Carefully selected patients with alcoholic liver disease, including those with severe alcoholic hepatitis, will have similar short-term and long-term outcomes when compared with other indications for liver transplant.
- Common causes of death late after liver transplantation in patients with alcoholic liver disease include cardiovascular disease and de novo head and neck malignancies, especially among those who smoke.

INTRODUCTION

Excessive chronic alcohol consumption is a common health care problem around the world. It results in high morbidity and mortality that stems not only from alcohol's effects on the liver, but the risk it poses to the health of other organ systems, as well as increased risk for accidents and violence-related deaths.

From a liver transplant standpoint, end-stage liver disease secondary to alcoholic cirrhosis is the second most frequent indication for liver transplantation in the United States and Europe, only surpassed by chronic hepatitis C (HCV). Posttransplant outcomes for most patients with alcoholic liver disease are comparable to those of other etiologies; however, patients with alcoholic liver disease have increased graft loss and

The authors have nothing to disclose.
[a] Division of Gastroenterology, Hepatology and Nutrition, University of Utah School of Medicine, 30 North 1900 East, SOM 4R118, Salt Lake City, UT 84132, USA; [b] Intermountain Transplant Center, Intermountain Medical Center, 5169 South Cottonwood Street, Suite 320, Murray, UT 84107, USA
* Corresponding author.
E-mail address: michael.charlton@imail.org

Clin Liver Dis 20 (2016) 521–534
http://dx.doi.org/10.1016/j.cld.2016.02.009
1089-3261/16/$ – see front matter © 2016 Elsevier Inc. All rights reserved.
liver.theclinics.com

mortality if they return to heavy alcohol use. Also, the causes of death seem to differ from that of other causes of liver transplantation, with an increased frequency of cardiovascular disease and de novo malignancies.

Although still controversial, liver transplantation has been successful in saving the lives of very select patients with severe alcoholic hepatitis (AH) not responding to medical therapy, and in the future might become another accepted indication for transplantation.

Although patients with alcoholic liver disease pose specific challenges in the pre-transplant and posttransplant setting, they can be overall good candidates for trans-plantation with excellent long-term outcomes.

EPIDEMIOLOGY OF ALCOHOL USE AND ALCOHOLIC LIVER DISEASE

Chronic excessive alcohol use is a major cause of preventable morbidity and mortality around the world. The World Health Organization (WHO) estimates that approximately 3.3 million deaths worldwide in 2012 were associated with alcohol misuse.[1] Not only does chronic alcohol misuse lead to organ damage, it can also lead to increased risk of accidents and violence resulting in morbidity and mortality. The negative effects of alcohol use disproportionately affect the young.

Data from WHO show 9% of all deaths in people aged 15 to 29 years were related to alcohol use. This amounts to approximately 320,000 deaths worldwide. In the United States, as of 2010, an estimated 140 million adults drink alcohol, with a prevalence of alcohol use disorder of 7.4% (10.7% in men and 4.2% of women).[1] Almost 25% of adult drinkers reported heavy episodic alcohol use (defined as drinking 60 g of alcohol or more on at least one occasion in the previous 30 days). The annual per capita alcohol consumption among American adults is 13.6 L in men and 4.9 L in women. The age-standardized death rate per 100,000 population for alcoholic cirrhosis in men is 14.9 and 7.1 for women.[1,2]

Excessive alcohol consumption is the third leading cause of preventable death in the United States, accounting for almost 90,000 deaths per year from 2006 to 2010.[3] Recent estimates suggest that approximately 18,000 Americans died from alcoholic liver disease in 2013 alone.[4]

The health consequences of alcohol drinking vary according to extent and method of usage, and also with environmental and genetic factors. Chronic alcohol use can lead to liver cirrhosis and is associated with increased risk of hepatocellular carci-noma. In Europe, 11% of deaths in men and 1.8% in women were attributable to excessive alcohol use.[2,5]

In 2010, liver cirrhosis accounted for almost 500,000 deaths worldwide, and approx-imately 15 million disability-adjusted life years (DALYs). Approximately 82,000 deaths (approximately 14,000 female and 66,000 male) and 2 million DALYs were due to alcohol-induced liver cancer.[6-9] The relevance of alcohol consumption on liver-related mortality is strongly supported by recent data that demonstrate a close rela-tionship between the standardized death rate of chronic liver disease and cirrhosis and overall alcohol consumption.[10] Other supporting data on the relationship between alcohol and mortality include the fact that reductions in alcohol consumption in most countries are followed by a decrease in cirrhosis-related mortality.

In North America, Australia, and parts of southern Europe, alcohol consumption has decreased in recent years, with associated declines in liver-related mortality.[11-14]

In the recent past, there has been a change in the nomenclature of alcohol-related health problems. Alcohol abuse and alcohol dependence, as defined in the Diagnostic and Statistical Manual of Mental Disorders, Fourth Edition (DSM-IV) have been substituted by the encompassing term alcohol use disorder, which is defined as a problematic pattern of alcohol use leading to clinically significant impairment or distress as described in DSM-5 (**Box 1**).[15]

LIVER TRANSPLANTATION AND ALCOHOLIC LIVER DISEASE

Alcoholic liver disease is a major indication for liver transplantation worldwide. In the United States and Europe, alcoholic liver cirrhosis is the second most common indication for liver transplantation, behind only chronic HCV. Alcoholic liver disease accounts for approximately 40% of primary liver transplants in Europe, and approximately 20% in the United States.[16–18]

In a recent analysis of the United Network for Organ Sharing database in the United States from 1987 to 2013, the percentage of liver transplants performed for alcoholic liver cirrhosis has varied from 17.7% in the cohort transplanted from 2007 to 2013, to a

---

Box 1
Current definition of alcohol use disorder as per the Diagnostic and Statistical Manual of Mental Disorders, Fifth Edition

Alcohol use disorder is defined as a problematic pattern of alcohol use leading to clinically significant impairment or distress, as manifested by at least 2 of the following, occurring within a 12-month period:

1. Alcohol is often taken in larger amounts for over a longer period than was intended.
2. There is a persistent desire or unsuccessful efforts to cut down or control alcohol use.
3. A great deal of time is spent in activities necessary to obtain alcohol, use alcohol, or recover from its effects.
4. Craving, or a stronger desire or urge to use alcohol.
5. Recurrent alcohol use resulting in a failure to fulfill major role obligations at work, school, or home.
6. Continued alcohol use despite having persistent or recurrent social or interpersonal problems caused or exacerbated by the effects of alcohol.
7. Important social, occupational, or recreational activities are given up or reduced because of alcohol use.
8. Recurrent alcohol use in situations in which it is physically hazardous.
9. Alcohol use is continued despite knowledge of having a persistent or recurrent physical or psychological problem that is likely to have been caused or exacerbated by alcohol.
10. Tolerance, as defined by either of the following:
    a. A need for markedly increased amounts of alcohol to achieve intoxication or desired effect.
    b. A markedly diminished effect with continued use of the same amount of alcohol.
11. Withdrawal, as manifested by either of the following:
    a. The characteristic withdrawal syndrome for alcohol.
    b. Alcohol (or a closely related substance, such as a benzodiazepine) is taken to relieve or avoid withdrawal symptoms.

The severity of the alcohol use disorder is provided by the number of items fulfilled, such that mild alcohol use disorder is characterized by 2 to 3 of the listed features, moderate when 4 or 5 features are present, and severe when 6 or more of the listed items are present.

From American Psychiatric Association. Alcohol-related disorders. In: American Psychiatric Association, editor. Diagnostic and statistical manual of mental disorders. 5th edition. Washington, DC: American Psychiatric Publishing; 2013. p. 490; with permission.

high of 23.1% in the cohort transplanted between 1994 and 2000.[18] The frequency of HCV as an indication for liver transplantation has been declining in the United States, whereas alcoholic liver cirrhosis and nonalcoholic fatty liver disease are on the rise, with trajectory for alcoholic liver disease exceeding that of nonalcoholic liver disease (**Fig. 1**). An inevitable consequence of the advent of highly effective and well-tolerated treatments for HCV infection will be further declines in HCV as an indication for liver transplantation, with relatively increased frequency of alcoholic liver disease as an indication.

ALCOHOLIC LIVER DISEASE IN THE PRETRANSPLANT PERIOD

Patients suffering from end-stage alcoholic liver disease who require liver transplantation present a special challenge to the transplant teams, as they have a high prevalence of alcohol-related comorbidities, such as protein-energy malnutrition, chronic anemia, neurologic disorders, kidney dysfunction, heart disease, and psychiatric comorbidities, including substance abuse.[19,20] The risk of relapse of alcohol use disorder following liver transplantation, with potential associated liver damage, is a specific risk that mandates careful evaluation and management strategies.[19]

In general, the indications and contraindications for liver transplantation in patients with end-stage liver disease related to alcohol use are similar to that of other causes. There are, however, specific considerations that need to be addressed in these patients. A detailed history of alcohol use and its consequences needs to be obtained at the time of evaluation, as well as a history of the use of other substances, such as tobacco, opioid analgesics, and illicit/recreational drugs. Simple, standardized questionnaires can be used in daily clinical practice to screen for chronic excessive alcohol use in patients undergoing transplant evaluation regardless of liver disease etiology. These include the CAGE questions (answered as yes/no, with 2 or more yes answers concerning for excessive alcohol consumption), as well as WHO's Alcohol Use Disorders Identification Test (AUDIT) questionnaire, which consists of 10 questions and can be self-administered.[21,22] This is considered the single best

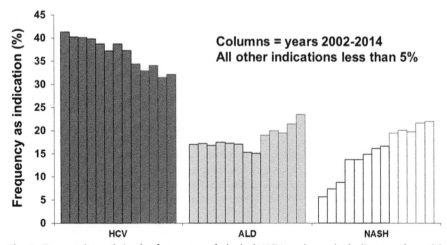

Fig. 1. Temporal trends in the frequency of alcohol, HCV, and nonalcoholic steatohepatitis (NASH) as indications for liver transplantation in the United States are shown. NASH and 50% of cryptogenic cirrhosis have been combined to account for the high frequency of NASH as a cause of cryptogenic cirrhosis. ALD, alcoholic liver disease. (*Data from* Scientific Registry of Transplant Recipients (SRTR). Available at: www.optn.transplant.hrsa.gov.)

instrument to systematically recognize and diagnose excessive chronic alcohol consumption. A free copy of the form can be downloaded from the National Institute on Alcohol Abuse and Alcoholism Web site (audit online; http://pubs.niaaa.nih.gov/publications/Audit.pdf).

In 1997, a group of American liver transplant physicians developed a consensus for the indications of liver transplantation and the minimal criteria required for placing patients on the transplant list. One of their recommendations was to require a minimum period of abstinence of 6 months in patients with alcoholic liver disease (the so-called "6-month rule"). The rationale behind this recommendation was to allow the full benefits of alcohol abstinence on liver function and its potential recovery, as it has been observed that typically patients will improve within 3 to 6 months of sobriety.[23,24] Currently, the American Association for the Study of Liver Diseases recommends that patients with alcoholic cirrhosis who continue to have significant liver dysfunction despite 6 months of sobriety, should be considered and evaluated for liver transplantation.[25] Most transplant programs in North America follow the 6-month rule of sobriety in patients with alcoholic liver disease; however, this period of abstinence is only a weak predictor of posttransplant drinking.[26,27] Many patients with chronic alcohol use will relapse after transplant despite 6 months of pretransplant sobriety.[28] There are data to suggest that abstinence might not be secure until after 5 years of sobriety.[29]

Rigid adherence to the 6-month rule may result in hazardous and unnecessary delays in listing patients with severe alcoholic liver disease who are otherwise good candidates for liver transplantation, including those with AH, who have a low risk of relapse of alcohol use disorder after transplantation. Experiences from Europe, specifically with regard to transplanting patients with severe AH, have demonstrated that in the appropriate setting, shorter periods of abstinence are not necessarily associated with return to drinking after transplantation.[30] Consensus conferences from the United Kingdom and France published in 2006 did not recommend a fixed interval of alcohol abstinence in patients with alcoholic liver disease in need of a liver transplant.[31,32] An Italian consensus on liver transplantation in patients with alcoholic liver disease recommended a 6-month abstinence period for patients with Model for End-Stage Liver Disease (MELD) score less than 19, a 3-month period was acceptable for selected patients with higher MELD scores, and in patients with severe AH not responding to medical management, no minimum period of sobriety is required before transplantation.[33]

Psychiatrists, psychologists, social workers, and addiction specialists are all essential in the multidisciplinary evaluation of patients with alcoholic liver disease undergoing pretransplant evaluation. The information gathered will help the multidisciplinary team assess the transplant candidacy of these patients, as well as to establish a management plan to treat the alcohol addiction before and after liver transplantation, so as to increase the success of liver transplantation in the individual patient.

One of the key issues to address during the pretransplant evaluation of candidates with alcoholic liver disease is the individual's risk of posttransplant relapse of alcohol use disorder. Currently, there is no single instrument that will provide a precise estimate of the risk of relapse after liver transplantation in patients with alcoholic liver disease; however, there are certain factors that suggest a favorable outcome. These include the following:

1. Patient acknowledgment of alcohol addiction
2. A social support system (particularly a spouse)
3. Paid employment
4. A home

5. Indicators of social integration
6. Activities to replace drinking in daily life
7. Support of a "rehabilitation relationship"
8. A source of improved self-esteem or of hope for the future
9. Identification by the patient of the negative consequences of return to drinking

In general, patients with less severe drinking patterns, previously known as alcohol abuse, seem to be at lower risk of recidivism after liver transplantation compared with patients with more severe drinking patterns, previously known as alcohol dependence.[34,35]

In a recent systematic review, Rustad and colleagues[36] reported that prospective studies document that a short period of pretransplant sobriety (less than 3–6 months) is a significant predictor of time to first drink and time to binge use. Presence of psychiatric comorbidity, high score on the standardized High-risk Alcoholism Relapse Scale, and diagnosis of alcohol dependence (by DSM-IV criteria) are all predictive of posttransplant alcohol relapse. Also, certain pretransplant variables, such as family history of alcoholism, can discriminate between recipients that become complete abstainers and those who go back to drinking.

Many transplant centers apply the Psychosocial Assessment of Candidacy for Transplantation scale as part of their evaluation process. This instrument is used to assess a candidate's social support, psychological health, lifestyle factors, and understanding of the transplant process, including posttransplant follow-up. Alcohol and substance use are only part of this scale. Patients are then classified into low, moderate, or high risk for relapse, helping to guide decision-making by the selection committee. Candidates with intermediate risk for alcohol recidivism are commonly referred to rehabilitation treatment (intensive outpatient vs inpatient rehabilitation) before consideration for liver transplantation, whereas those in the low-risk category can be listed immediately and those at high risk for relapse are typically deferred or denied listing.[37,38]

A more recent instrument to help with the psychosocial evaluation of the transplant candidate is the Stanford Integrated Psychosocial Assessment for Transplantation (SIPAT). Strengths of the SIPAT include the standardization of the evaluation process and its ability to identify subjects who are at risk for negative psychosocial outcomes after transplantation, so as to allow for the development of interventions directed at improving the patient's candidacy. The use of this instrument allows the assessment of psychosocial factors that appear to better predict patient adherence and graft survival. A total of 18 risk factors are divided into 4 domains, including patient readiness, social support, psychological stability, and substance abuse. Based on a composite score of all these domains, patients are classified as excellent, good, minimally acceptable, high risk, or poor candidates for transplantation.[39] However, the decision to list a transplant candidate will ultimately rely on the multidisciplinary selection committee.

After the patient has been formally listed for liver transplantation, it is important to ask about alcohol use relapse, and obtain information not only from the patient, but also from the social support network to confirm sobriety. Many patients will also be tested for alcohol use through indirect markers such as gamma glutamyl transferase or carbohydrate-deficient transferrin; or by direct markers such as blood ethanol or methanol levels, urine ethyl glucuronide, or ethyl sulfate and phosphatidyl ethanol.[40] The short-term window for positivity after the last heavy alcohol consumption limits the utility of these tests in clinical practice. Typically blood alcohol levels and methanol levels will be positive only for a few hours after last consumption, whereas urine ethyl glucuronide or ethyl sulfate can be positive 4 to 5 days after the last alcohol use.[41] Hair analysis for ethyl glucuronide can be useful in this setting, as the metabolite will be detectable up to 1 month after last alcohol use.[42] However, hair analysis is not widely available. Wait-listed patients who relapse with alcohol use should receive further chemical dependency counseling and should be made temporarily inactive on the transplant waitlist or potentially delisted until abstinence is achieved and sustained.

POSTTRANSPLANT OUTCOMES IN ALCOHOLIC LIVER DISEASE

Survival in patients transplanted for alcoholic liver disease is comparable to that of other etiologies, and even better than the long-term survival observed in patients transplanted for HCV.[43] In large transplant registries from Europe and the United States, the 1-year, 3-year, and 5-year patient survival ranges from 81% to 92%, 78% to 86%, and 73% to 86%, respectively.[16,17] However, emerging data suggest patients with alcoholic liver disease with posttransplant relapses have a reduced survival, more progressive liver injury, and even episodes of AH and cirrhosis.[44–47]

Alcohol use relapse is reported in 10% to 60% of liver transplant recipients transplanted for alcoholic liver disease.[35,48–50] This wide variation is probably a consequence of different definitions of relapse. Some groups have defined relapse as any alcohol use after transplantation, whereas others define it as patients with "harmful drinking" (2 or more alcohol drinks per day), which is reported in approximately 15% to 20% of patients.[51–53]

In a prospective analysis of 208 liver transplants in patients with alcoholic liver disease followed for 9 years, DiMartini and colleagues[52] were able to assess posttransplant alcohol drinking patterns in detail. Fifty-one percent of the recipients never returned to drinking. Among the 95 nonabstainers, 4 patterns of drinking were described: (1) most drank small amounts of alcohol infrequently (n = 55, 28.6%), (2) others had early onset of moderate alcohol consumption that decreased over time (n = 13, 6.4%), (3) others had later onset moderate use that increased over time (n = 15, 7.9%), and (4) a minority had an early onset of heavy alcohol use that increased over time (n = 12, 5.8%).[52] Interestingly, patients in groups 2 and 4, with early and heavier alcohol use than the other patients, were more likely to have rejection or steatohepatitis on liver biopsy and more likely to experience graft failure; and all recipients who died from recurrent alcoholic liver disease were in these groups. Certain elements of the alcohol history allowed the identification of drinkers compared with abstainers after liver transplantation. These variables included a formal diagnosis of alcohol dependence, short length of sobriety, family history of alcoholism, and use of other substances. Ideally, early identification of the trajectory of alcohol use in the posttransplant period will allow transplant teams to target preventive and interventional treatment to those individuals identified as high risk for alcohol misuse. It is important to bear in mind that graft failure due to posttransplant relapsing alcohol use is highly unusual, much less frequent than graft loss due to recurrence of HCV, for example.

In a retrospective review of 300 patients transplanted for alcoholic liver disease, Rice and colleagues[47] identified 48 recipients (16%) who had alcohol use that came to the attention of the clinician. Of these recipients, a single episode was identified in 10 (21%), intermittent relapses were noted in 22 (46%), and continuous heavy drinking was seen in 16 (33%). This last pattern of drinking was associated with an almost threefold increased rate of graft loss when compared with abstainers. When comparing histopathologic features of the allograft, patients who returned to drinking, compared with those who maintained abstinence, were more likely to have significant steatosis, steatohepatitis, and advanced fibrosis (stage $\geq$3).[47]

More recently, Dumortier and colleagues[54] performed a retrospective analysis of 712 patients transplanted for alcoholic cirrhosis in 3 centers in France. After a mean follow-up of 9 years, 128 patients (18%) experienced severe alcoholic relapse (defined as mean alcohol consumption >20 g per day in women or >30 g per day in men, for at least 6 months). Relapse was observed a median of 25 months after transplantation (range 4–157 months). Among this group, recurrent alcoholic cirrhosis was identified in 41 recipients (32%, or 6% of the entire group), a median of 5 years after transplantation (range 1.8–13.9 years) and 4 years after alcohol relapse (range 1.2–11.5 years). Recurrent alcoholic cirrhosis was associated with younger age at transplantation and a shorter period of pretransplant sobriety. Finally, 1-year, 5-year, 10-year, and 15-year patient survival was 100%, 88%, 50%, and 21%, respectively, for patients with recurrent alcoholic cirrhosis compared with 100%, 89%, 70%, and 41%, respectively, for patients without recurrence (P<.001). A third of the patients with severe alcohol relapse develop cirrhosis within 5 years of transplantation, which is similar to HCV recurrence and represents an accelerated natural history of alcoholic liver disease after transplantation. In line with what has been described in posttransplant HCV, the long-term survival of patients with recurrent alcoholic cirrhosis is quite poor, with 10-year survival of 50% and 15-year survival of 21%. Patient death in this group was associated with graft failure, and to other complications of alcohol use, such as de novo extrahepatic malignancies, cardiovascular disease, and suicide. These results emphasize the importance of assessing alcohol use after transplantation and providing appropriate addiction management once identified, so as to avoid the negative long-term consequences of alcohol recidivism.

Causes of death after transplantation in patients with alcoholic liver disease seem to differ compared with those of other etiologies, specifically with regard to the increased frequency of cardiovascular disease and de novo malignancies.[55–58] Most of the new-onset malignancies are concentrated within the respiratory and digestive tracts. Cigarette smoking is a well-established risk factor for these types of cancers, as well as for cardiovascular disease. It has been postulated that the increased frequency of these as a cause of death among recipients transplanted for alcoholic liver disease is due to the high prevalence of tobacco use among these patients.[59] Indeed, many of these patients quickly go back to smoking after transplantation.[60] These patients should be strongly encouraged to quit tobacco and adhere to a smoke-free lifestyle to decrease the risk of cardiovascular disease and de novo cancer.

LIVER TRANSPLANTATION IN ALCOHOLIC HEPATITIS

AH is a distinct clinical syndrome seen in patients with chronic excessive alcohol use characterized by worsening jaundice, mild to moderate elevation in liver enzymes, coagulopathy, and hepatic encephalopathy. At times it can present as acute-on-chronic liver failure.[61,62]

AH has significant morbidity and mortality, as documented both in Europe and the United States.[63,64] In the United States, there were 57,000 hospitalizations for AH in 2007, accounting for 0.7% of all admissions with an inpatient mortality of 7% to 15%.[63,64] In its severe form, AH can have a mortality of 30% to 50% at 3 months and up to 70% at 6 months, especially when associated with acute kidney injury.[65,66] Most of these patients already have liver cirrhosis on biopsy.[67]

The currently available treatment options for severe AH include prednisone and pentoxifylline.[5,25,61,62,66] However, their benefit has been questioned by the results of a recent randomized controlled trial from the United Kingdom of 1100 patients with severe AH in which no obvious 28-day, 90-day, and 1-year survival advantage was apparent when compared with placebo.[68] In other studies, medical therapy has been shown to decrease short-term mortality by 50%, still leaving a substantial number of patients without any real options for recovery. As most transplant centers in the United States require a 6-month alcohol abstinence period before transplantation, most patients with severe AH are effectively excluded from this life-saving intervention. However, in the few instances when they have been transplanted, their outcomes are comparable to those seen in patients transplanted for liver cirrhosis.

Singal and colleagues[69] performed a retrospective review of the United Network for Organ Sharing database (2004–2010) of adults undergoing liver transplantation for a listing diagnosis of AH (n = 59). They were matched for age, gender, ethnicity, MELD score, donor risk index, and year of transplantation with patients transplanted for a diagnosis of alcoholic cirrhosis. Five-year graft and patient survival of patients with AH or alcoholic cirrhosis were 75% and 73% (P = .97) and 80% and 78% (P = .90), respectively. After adjusting for other variables, there was no impact of the etiology of liver disease (AH vs alcoholic cirrhosis) on graft and patient survival. The causes of graft loss and patient mortality were similar in the 2 groups, and were not alcohol-related in any patient. Two single-center retrospective studies based on explant histopathology also demonstrated similar patient survival regardless of the presence or absence of AH on the explanted liver.[70,71]

Because the French consensus recommendations do not advocate for a specific length of sobriety before liver transplantation, a multicenter prospective trial of early liver transplantation in patients with severe AH not responding to steroid therapy was performed in Europe and reported in 2011.[30] A total of 26 patients from 7 centers in France and Belgium with severe AH at high risk of death (median MELD 34) were selected and placed on the list for a liver transplant within a median of 13 days after nonresponse to medical therapy with prednisolone. Selection required full agreement among all members of the multidisciplinary team caring for these patients. The cumulative 6-month survival rate was higher among patients who received early transplantation than among those who did not (77% vs 23%, P<.001). This benefit of early transplantation was maintained through 2 years of follow-up (hazard ratio 6.08; P = .004). Fewer than 2% of patients admitted for an episode of severe AH were selected. The centers used 3% of available grafts for this indication. Only 3 recipients resumed drinking alcohol, none of them within 2 years after transplantation. More data on the safety and efficacy of liver transplantation in patients with severe AH are needed before this practice can be generalized to other centers; however, the door is now open for very select patients with a first episode of AH to be considered for liver transplantation if not responding to usual medical care.

One of the concerns of transplanting patients with AH is how the public would view liver transplantation for these patients. There is already a generally negative perception of liver transplantation for alcoholics by the public. Studies have shown that the public and even health care providers view organ allocation to patients with alcoholic liver disease (perceived as a self-inflicted disease) less favorably than those with acquired or inherited liver diseases.[72–74] In an effort to understand the public views on liver transplantation for patients with alcoholic liver disease and specifically early transplantation for those with severe AH, Stroh and colleagues[75] conducted on online survey among 500 participants through a crowdsourcing marketplace. The survey measured attitudes on liver transplantation in general, and on early transplant for patients with AH specifically, in addition to measuring responses to 9 vignettes describing fictional candidates with alcoholic hepatitis. Most respondents (82%, n = 410) were at least neutral toward early transplantation for these patients. Only a minority (26%) indicated that transplantation in these patients would make them hesitant to donate their organs. Middle-aged patients with good social support and financial stability were viewed most favorably. Age was considered the most important selection factor and financial stability the least important factor. These results indicate early liver transplantation for carefully selected patients with acute AH may not be as controversial to the public as previously believed.

SUMMARY

Excessive chronic alcohol consumption is a common health care problem around the world, with significant morbidity and mortality. End-stage liver disease secondary to alcoholic cirrhosis is the second most frequent cause for liver transplantation in the United States and Europe. Posttransplant outcomes for most patients with alcoholic liver disease are comparable to those of other etiologies; however, patients with alcoholic liver disease have increased graft loss and mortality if they return to heavy alcohol use. Also, the causes of death seem to differ from that of other etiologies of liver transplantation, with an increased frequency of cardiovascular disease and de novo malignancies.

Although still controversial, liver transplantation has been successful in saving the lives of very select patients with severe AH not responding to medical therapy, and in the future might become another indication for transplantation.

Although patients with alcoholic liver disease pose specific challenges in the pretransplant and posttransplant settings, they are overall good candidates for transplantation with excellent long-term outcomes.

REFERENCES

1. WHO. Global status report on alcohol and health 2014. Geneva, Switzerland: WHO; 2014. Available at: http://www.who.int/substance_abuse/publications/global_alcohol_report/en/.
2. Schwartz JM, Reinus JF. Prevalence and natural history of alcoholic liver disease. Clin Liver Dis 2012;16:659–66.
3. CDC. Alcohol related disease impact (ARDI). Centers for Disease Control and Prevention; 2013. Available at. http://nccd.cdc.gov/DPH_ARDI/Default.aspx.
4. Udompap P, Kim D, Kim WR. Current and future burden of chronic nonmalignant liver disease. Clin Gastroenterol Hepatol 2015;13:2031–41.
5. European Association for the Study of Liver. EASL clinical practical guidelines: management of alcoholic liver disease. J Hepatol 2012;57:399–420.
6. Lozano R, Naghavi M, Foreman K, et al. Global and regional mortality from 235 causes of death for 20 age groups in 1990 and 2010: a systematic analysis for the Global Burden of Disease Study 2010. Lancet 2012;380: 2095–128.
7. Mathurin P, Bataller R. Trends in the management and burden of alcoholic liver disease. J Hepatol 2015;62:S38–46.
8. Murray CJ, Vos T, Lozano R, et al. Disability-adjusted life years (DALYs) for 291 diseases and injuries in 21 regions, 1990-2010: a systematic analysis for the Global Burden of Disease Study 2010. Lancet 2012;380:2197–223.
9. Rehm J, Samokhvalov AV, Shield KD. Global burden of alcoholic liver diseases. J Hepatol 2013;59:160–8.
10. Jewell J, Sheron N. Trends in European liver death rates: implications for alcohol policy. Clin Med 2010;10:259–63.
11. Bosetti C, Levi F, Lucchini F, et al. Worldwide mortality from cirrhosis: an update to 2002. J Hepatol 2007;46:827–39.

12. Corrao G, Ferrari P, Zambon A, et al. Trends of liver cirrhosis mortality in Europe, 1970-1989: age-period-cohort analysis and changing alcohol consumption. Int J Epidemiol 1997;26:100–9.
13. Leon DA, Shkolnikov VM, McKee M. Alcohol and Russian mortality: a continuing crisis. Addiction 2009;104:1630–6.
14. Ramstedt M. Per capita alcohol consumption and liver cirrhosis mortality in 14 European countries. Addiction 2001;96(Suppl 1):S19–33.
15. American Psychiatric Association. Alcohol-related disorders. In: American Psychiatric Association, editor. Diagnostic and statistical manual of mental disorders. 5th edition. Washington, DC: American Psychiatric Publishing; 2013. p. 490–503.
16. Burra P, Senzolo M, Adam R, et al. Liver transplantation for alcoholic liver disease in Europe: a study from the ELTR (European liver transplant registry). Am J Transplant 2010;10:138–48.
17. Singal AK, Guturu P, Hmoud B, et al. Evolving frequency and outcomes of liver transplantation based on etiology of liver disease. Transplantation 2013;95: 755–60.
18. Stepanova M, Wai H, Saab S, et al. The portrait of an adult liver transplant recipient in the United States from 1987 to 2013. JAMA Intern Med 2014;174:1407–9.
19. Leong J, Im GY. Evaluation and selection of the patient with alcoholic liver disease for liver transplant. Clin Liver Dis 2012;16:851–63.
20. Singal AK, Charlton MR. Nutrition in alcoholic liver disease. Clin Liver Dis 2012; 16:805–26.
21. Ewing JA. Detecting alcoholism. The CAGE questionnaire. JAMA 1984;252: 1905–7.
22. Saunders JB, Aasland OG, Babor TF, et al. Development of the alcohol use disorders identification test (AUDIT): WHO collaborative project on early detection of persons with harmful alcohol consumption–II. Addiction 1993;88:791–804.
23. Hoofnagle JH, Kresina T, Fuller RK, et al. Liver transplantation for alcoholic liver disease: executive statement and recommendations. Summary of a National Institutes of Health workshop held December 6-7, 1996, Bethesda, Maryland. Liver Transpl Surg 1997;3:347–50.
24. Lucey MR. Issues in selection for and outcome of liver transplantation in patients with alcoholic liver disease. Liver Transpl Surg 1997;3:227–30.
25. O'Shea RS, Dasarathy S, McCullough AJ, Practice Guideline Committee of the American Association for the Study of Liver Diseases, Practice Parameters Committee of the American College of Gastroenterology. Alcoholic liver disease. Hepatology 2010;51:307–28.
26. Everhart JE, Beresford TP. Liver transplantation for alcoholic liver disease: a survey of transplantation programs in the United States. Liver Transpl Surg 1997;3: 220–6.
27. Yates WR, Martin M, LaBrecque D, et al. A model to examine the validity of the 6-month abstinence criterion for liver transplantation. Alcohol Clin Exp Res 1998;22:513–7.
28. Karim Z, Intaraprasong P, Scudamore CH, et al. Predictors of relapse to significant alcohol drinking after liver transplantation. Can J Gastroenterol 2010;24: 245–50.
29. Vanlemmens C, Di Martino V, Milan C, et al. Immediate listing for liver transplantation versus standard care for Child-Pugh stage B alcoholic cirrhosis: a randomized trial. Ann Intern Med 2009;150:153–61.
30. Mathurin P, Moreno C, Samuel D, et al. Early liver transplantation for severe alcoholic hepatitis. N Engl J Med 2011;365:1790–800.

31. Bathgate AJ, Units UKLT. Recommendations for alcohol-related liver disease. Lancet 2006;367:2045–6.
32. Webb K, Shepherd L, Day E, et al. Transplantation for alcoholic liver disease: report of a consensus meeting. Liver Transpl 2006;12:301–5.
33. Testino G, Burra P, Bonino F, et al. Acute alcoholic hepatitis, end stage alcoholic liver disease and liver transplantation: an Italian position statement. World J Gastroenterol 2014;20:14642–51.
34. Beresford TP. Psychiatric assessment of alcoholic candidates for liver transplantation. In: Lucey M, Merion RM, Beresford TP, editors. Liver transplantation and the alcoholic patient. Cambridge (United Kingdom): Cambridge University Press; 1994. p. 29–49.
35. Lucey MR. Liver transplantation for alcoholic liver disease. Nat Rev Gastroenterol Hepatol 2014;11:300–7.
36. Rustad JK, Stern TA, Prabhakar M, et al. Risk factors for alcohol relapse following orthotopic liver transplantation: a systematic review. Psychosomatics 2015;56: 21–35.
37. Olbrisch ME, Levenson JL. Liver transplantation for alcoholic cirrhosis. JAMA 1989;261:2958.
38. Singal AK, Chaha KS, Rasheed K, et al. Liver transplantation in alcoholic liver disease: current status and controversies. World J Gastroenterol 2013;19: 5953–63.
39. Maldonado JR, Dubois HC, David EE, et al. The Stanford Integrated Psychosocial Assessment for Transplantation (SIPAT): a new tool for the psychosocial evaluation of pre-transplant candidates. Psychosomatics 2012;53:123–32.
40. Allen JP, Wurst FM, Thon N, et al. Assessing the drinking status of liver transplant patients with alcoholic liver disease. Liver Transpl 2013;19:369–76.
41. Staufer K, Andresen H, Vettorazzi E, et al. Urinary ethyl glucuronide as a novel screening tool in patients pre- and post-liver transplantation improves detection of alcohol consumption. Hepatology 2011;54:1640–9.
42. Sterneck M, Yegles M, Rothkirch von G, et al. Determination of ethyl glucuronide in hair improves evaluation of long-term alcohol abstention in liver transplant candidates. Liver Int 2014;34:469–76.
43. Gaglio PJ Jr, Gaglio PJ Sr. Complications in patients with alcohol-associated liver disease who undergo liver transplantation. Clin Liver Dis 2012;16:865–75.
44. Conjeevaram HS, Hart J, Lissoos TW, et al. Rapidly progressive liver injury and fatal alcoholic hepatitis occurring after liver transplantation in alcoholic patients. Transplantation 1999;67:1562–8.
45. Cuadrado A, Fabrega E, Casafont F, et al. Alcohol recidivism impairs long-term patient survival after orthotopic liver transplantation for alcoholic liver disease. Liver Transpl 2005;11:420–6.
46. Pfitzmann R, Schwenzer J, Rayes N, et al. Long-term survival and predictors of relapse after orthotopic liver transplantation for alcoholic liver disease. Liver Transpl 2007;13:197–205.
47. Rice JP, Eickhoff J, Agni R, et al. Abusive drinking after liver transplantation is associated with allograft loss and advanced allograft fibrosis. Liver Transpl 2013;19:1377–86.
48. Lucey MR, Carr K, Beresford TP, et al. Alcohol use after liver transplantation in alcoholics: a clinical cohort follow-up study. Hepatology 1997;25:1223–7.
49. Newton SE. Recidivism and return to work posttransplant. Recipients with substance abuse histories. J Subst Abuse Treat 1999;17:103–8.

50. Tandon P, Goodman KJ, Ma MM, et al. A shorter duration of pre-transplant absti-nence predicts problem drinking after liver transplantation. Am J Gastroenterol 2009;104:1700–6.
51. DiMartini A, Day N, Dew MA, et al. Alcohol consumption patterns and predictors of use following liver transplantation for alcoholic liver disease. Liver Transpl 2006;12:813–20.
52. DiMartini A, Dew MA, Day N, et al. Trajectories of alcohol consumption following liver transplantation. Am J Transplant 2010;10:2305–12.
53. Tang H, Boulton R, Gunson B, et al. Patterns of alcohol consumption after liver transplantation. Gut 1998;43:140–5.
54. Dumortier J, Dharancy S, Cannesson A, et al. Recurrent alcoholic cirrhosis in severe alcoholic relapse after liver transplantation: a frequent and serious compli-cation. Am J Gastroenterol 2015;110:1160–6 [quiz: 1167].
55. Bellamy CO, DiMartini AM, Ruppert K, et al. Liver transplantation for alcoholic cirrhosis: long term follow-up and impact of disease recurrence. Transplantation 2001;72:619–26.
56. Dumortier J, Guillaud O, Adham M, et al. Negative impact of de novo malig-nancies rather than alcohol relapse on survival after liver transplantation for alcoholic cirrhosis: a retrospective analysis of 305 patients in a single center. Am J Gastroenterol 2007;102:1032–41.
57. Saigal S, Norris S, Muiesan P, et al. Evidence of differential risk for posttransplan-tation malignancy based on pretransplantation cause in patients undergoing liver transplantation. Liver Transpl 2002;8:482–7.
58. Watt KD, Pedersen RA, Kremers WK, et al. Evolution of causes and risk factors for mortality post-liver transplant: results of the NIDDK long-term follow-up study. Am J Transplant 2010;10:1420–7.
59. Chak E, Saab S. Risk factors and incidence of de novo malignancy in liver trans-plant recipients: a systematic review. Liver Int 2010;30:1247–58.
60. DiMartini A, Javed L, Russell S, et al. Tobacco use following liver transplantation for alcoholic liver disease: an underestimated problem. Liver Transpl 2005;11: 679–83.
61. Singal AK, Kamath PS, Gores GJ, et al. Alcoholic hepatitis: current challenges and future directions. Clin Gastroenterol Hepatol 2014;12:555–64 [quiz: e531–552].
62. Sohail U, Satapathy SK. Diagnosis and management of alcoholic hepatitis. Clin Liver Dis 2012;16:717–36.
63. Liangpunsakul S. Clinical characteristics and mortality of hospitalized alcoholic hepatitis patients in the United States. J Clin Gastroenterol 2011;45:714–9.
64. Sandahl TD, Jepsen P, Thomsen KL, et al. Incidence and mortality of alcoholic hepatitis in Denmark 1999-2008: a nationwide population based cohort study. J Hepatol 2011;54:760–4.
65. Lucey MR, Mathurin P, Morgan TR. Alcoholic hepatitis. N Engl J Med 2009;360: 2758–69.
66. Mathurin P, Louvet A, Duhamel A, et al. Prednisolone with vs without pentoxifylline and survival of patients with severe alcoholic hepatitis: a randomized clinical trial. JAMA 2013;310:1033–41.
67. Altamirano J, Miquel R, Katoonizadeh A, et al. A histologic scoring system for prognosis of patients with alcoholic hepatitis. Gastroenterology 2014;146. 1231-9.e1–e6.
68. Thursz MR, Richardson P, Allison M, et al. Prednisolone or pentoxifylline for alco-holic hepatitis. N Engl J Med 2015;372:1619–28.

69. Singal AK, Bashar H, Anand BS, et al. Outcomes after liver transplantation for alcoholic hepatitis are similar to alcoholic cirrhosis: exploratory analysis from the UNOS database. Hepatology 2012;55:1398–405.

70. Tome S, Martinez-Rey C, Gonzalez-Quintela A, et al. Influence of superimposed alcoholic hepatitis on the outcome of liver transplantation for end-stage alcoholic liver disease. J Hepatol 2002;36:793–8.

71. Wells JT, Said A, Agni R, et al. The impact of acute alcoholic hepatitis in the explanted recipient liver on outcome after liver transplantation. Liver Transpl 2007;13:1728–35.

72. Wittenberg E, Goldie SJ, Fischhoff B, et al. Rationing decisions and individual responsibility for illness: are all lives equal? Med Decis Making 2003;23:194–211.

73. Neuberger J, Adams D, MacMaster P, et al. Assessing priorities for allocation of donor liver grafts: survey of public and clinicians. BMJ 1998;317:172–5.

74. Perut V, Conti F, Scatton O, et al. Might physicians be restricting access to liver transplantation for patients with alcoholic liver disease? J Hepatol 2009;51:707–14.

75. Stroh G, Rosell T, Dong F, et al. Early liver transplantation for patients with acute alcoholic hepatitis: public views and the effects on organ donation. Am J Transplant 2015;15:1598–604.

Nutrition and Alcoholic Liver Disease

Effects of Alcoholism on Nutrition, Effects of Nutrition on Alcoholic Liver Disease, and Nutritional Therapies for Alcoholic Liver Disease

Srinivasan Dasarathy, MD*

KEYWORDS

- Alcoholic liver disease • Malnutrition • Sarcopenia • Skeletal muscle loss
- Myostatin • Molecular pathways • Mitochondria • Reactive oxygen species

KEY POINTS

- Malnutrition is the most frequent complication in alcoholic liver disease, adversely affects the clinical consequences and includes loss of skeletal muscle mass or sarcopenia and perturbations in energy metabolism.
- Among the different etiologies of liver disease, malnutrition and sarcopenia are believed to be most severe in alcoholic liver disease.
- Very recent data show that alcohol is directly metabolized in the skeletal muscle and contributes to loss of muscle mass but the contribution of skeletal muscle ethanol metabolism to other organ injury is not known.
- There are no effective therapies for malnutrition and sarcopenia in alcoholic liver disease primarily because treatments used to date have focused on improved dietary intake and nutrient supplementation.
- Targeting myostatin, molecular signaling pathways that regulate protein synthesis and autophagy, and mitochondrial protective agents are exciting novel therapeutic strategies that are likely to reverse sarcopenia in ALD.

INTRODUCTION

The term malnutrition is defined as a condition when the body does not receive enough nutrition to maintain health. Malnutrition can also be defined as a loss of muscle and/or fat mass. In addition to skeletal muscle loss, another component

Dr S. Dasarathy's research has been funded in part by NIH RO1 DK 83414, R21 AA 022742, UO1 AA021893, and UO1DK061732.
Departments of Gastroenterology, Hepatology and Pathobiology, Lerner Research Institute, NE4 208, 9500 Euclid Avenue, Cleveland, OH 44195, USA
* Corresponding address: Department of Gastroenterology and Hepatology, Lerner Research Institute, NE4 208, 9500 Euclid Avenue, Cleveland, OH 44195.
E-mail address: dasaras@ccf.org

of malnutrition is an alteration in energy metabolism with accelerated starvation.[1,2] Malnutrition is the most frequent complication in liver disease and cirrhosis; however, there are no standardized definitions, which makes comparisons across studies difficult. It is necessary to accurately define nutritional status in alcoholic liver disease (ALD) so that published data are interpreted appropriately and the use of standardized terminology allows comparisons of results from different studies.[3] The term malnutrition has been used to define loss of body weight, muscle mass, fat mass, muscle strength, visceral protein levels, immune function, and poor oral intake of nutrients.[4–6] Each of these measures suffers from significant limitations. Visceral protein concentrations in blood including albumin, prealbumin, and retinol binding proteins have been used extensively but are truly measures of hepatic synthetic function.[4] Immune function is directly altered by alcohol and viral infection and cannot be truly considered measures of hepatic effects on the skeletal muscle or nutritional indices.[7] Anthropometric measures including skinfold thickness that measures fat mass and arm muscle area are used as nutritional indices but suffer from intraobserver and interobserver variability.[8] Nitrogen balance studies are difficult and suffer from imprecision in the clinical setting, long-term accurate dietary intake studies are difficult, and retrospective studies suffer from recall bias. The term malnutrition is increasingly used to refer to the phenotype of loss of skeletal muscle mass with/without fat loss and not dietary intake, digestion, and absorption of nutrients even though the latter contribute to muscle and fat loss and disordered energy metabolism.

The term sarcopenia refers to muscle loss in patients with chronic diseases.[2,9–11] Even though micronutrient deficiencies are common in alcoholic hepatitis and cirrhosis,[12,13] the focus of this article is on skeletal muscle loss and how it is integrated with the disordered energy metabolism in patients with ALD.

Most publications refer to malnutrition in cirrhosis and ALD without specifying if the effects are caused by sarcopenia, loss of fat mass, or a combination of both. Careful analyses of published studies show that sarcopenia is the major component of malnutrition[4,5,14,15] and liver injury and alcohol contribute to muscle loss. The role of nutritional deficiencies on progression of liver injury is not known. Myokines are proteins secreted by the skeletal muscle including interleukin-6 and -15, which may alter hepatic metabolism and fibrosis, but a muscle-liver axis has not yet been established.[16,17] This article focuses on prevalence and methods to quantify malnutrition, specifically sarcopenia; the mechanisms of muscle loss in ALD including the liver-muscle axis; and potential therapies including novel, molecular targeted treatments. The impact of disordered energy metabolism is discussed in the context of its contribution to sarcopenia. Micronutrient deficiencies including zinc are common in patients with ALD, and their impact on outcomes in ALD has been reviewed elsewhere and is not discussed in detail here.[12,13,18] The effect of different nutrient supplements on hepatic histology and liver function in ALD is also not discussed and the interested reader is referred to reviews published on this topic.[19,20] For more information on nutritional therapy for acute alcoholic hepatitis, see Phillips PK, Lucey MR: Acute Alcoholic Hepatitis – Therapy, in this issue.

PREVALENCE AND METHODS TO QUANTIFY MALNUTRITION IN ALCOHOLIC LIVER DISEASE

Malnutrition is present in 20% to 90% of patients with liver disease and sarcopenia in nearly 70% of these patients.[2,4,5,21,22] We have recently reported that the prevalence of alcoholic cirrhosis is likely to be the major form of liver disease in the

United States.[23] Therefore, malnutrition and its constituents, muscle loss and fat loss, are major clinical consequences that need to be managed. Different criteria have been used to define malnutrition but there is evolving consensus among hepatologists and transplant surgeons that the major determinant of outcome is skeletal muscle mass.[10,24] In addition to anthropometric measurements, lean body mass quantified by bioelectrical impedance analysis, dual-energy X-ray absorptiometry, and impedance plethysmography have also been used as a measure of skeletal muscle mass despite the recognized limitations of these techniques (**Table 1**).[25] Recently, imaging methods including ultrasonography, computed tomography, and MRI have been used to quantify skeletal muscle mass.[26,27] Skeletal muscle area determined from a single section at the third or fourth lumbar vertebra on computed tomography or MRI has been shown to reflect whole-body muscle mass.[26] Using these methods, patients with cirrhosis have lower muscle mass and fat mass compared with control subjects.[28,29] Even though most studies to date have included alcoholic cirrhosis as part of the cohort of patients with cirrhosis studied, there are no published data on differences in prevalence of sarcopenia defined by direct muscle mass measurements stratified by cause of cirrhosis.

Cirrhosis is a state of accelerated starvation that is defined not by appetite, but rather by the low respiratory quotient (RQ), which is the ratio of the oxygen consumed and carbon dioxide released.[28,30] Unlike that observed in healthy subjects, postprandial reduction in RQ occurs much earlier in patients with cirrhosis suggesting a more rapid fatty acid and amino acid oxidation as a source of energy.[30,31] Indirect calorimetry to define starvation and nutritional needs is not universally used even though hand-held, easy to use calorimeters are now available for clinical use.[28,32,33] Using these criteria, most patients with cirrhosis, at least in the hospitalized setting, have low RQ and the reduction in RQ is associated with sarcopenia providing the critical link between muscle and fat loss and disordered energy metabolism.

Although the clinical consequences of sarcopenia, the major component of malnutrition, are now well recognized, the other components of malnutrition, fat loss and altered whole-body energy use, are not as well understood and their contribution to clinical outcomes has not been evaluated but reduction in RQ has been reported to be accompanied by more severe muscle loss.[28] These observations suggest that accelerated use of fat is associated with muscle loss, but the mechanisms by which more rapid fatty acid oxidation results in sarcopenia are not well understood.

In the past, it was believed that patients with ALD have more severe malnutrition, using anthropometric and subjective global assessment criteria.[14,15,34] However, this has been questioned by others, who have reported no significant differences in the prevalence of malnutrition between alcoholic and nonalcoholic cirrhosis.[35,36] Concerns with interpretation of published data include the definition of and measures used to define malnutrition, the duration between the time alcohol was consumed last and the determination of nutritional indices, the severity of liver disease in different groups, and the contribution of other factors that result in progression of muscle and fat loss (**Box 1, Fig. 1**).[22,35,36]

CLINICAL CONSEQUENCES OF MALNUTRITION IN ALCOHOLIC LIVER DISEASE

Almost all patients with liver disease have some evidence of malnutrition, specifically sarcopenia.[21,37] Several factors contribute to malnutrition and sarcopenia in cirrhosis including ALD (**Boxes 2 and 3**). Even though the adverse impact of malnutrition on survival, quality of life, and development of other complications of cirrhosis has been well recognized,[1,2,38] recent data on the impact of sarcopenia have been much more

Table 1
Methods to quantify malnutrition in alcoholic liver disease

Assessment Tool	Advantages	Disadvantages
Anthropometry Skin fold thickness Limb circumference	Simple, inexpensive, easy to perform	Overinterpretation; muscle mass is not directly measured, bone size is assumed Interobserver and intraobserver variability makes reproducibility difficult Fat mass is measured but accuracy and precision not certain
Subjective global assessment	Simple, inexpensive, easy to use	Long questionnaire, modifications limit precision Main emphasis is on muscle mass Interobserver and intraobserver variability Fat and muscle mass contribute to score but muscle loss major factor
Grip strength	Objective, reproducible	Measures contractile strength and not muscle mass No measure of fat mass
Lean body mass Bioelecrical impedance analysis Dual-energy X-ray absorptiometry Impedance plethysmography	Objective, reproducible	Measures lean body/fat free mass, an indirect measure of muscle mass Dual-energy X-ray absorptiometry has risk of radiation, especially if used for repeated measures
Imaging methods Ultrasound Computed tomography abdomen MRI abdomen	Direct quantification of muscle and fat mass	Expensive Observer variability with ultrasound Radiation risk with computed tomography Single slices are an estimate of whole-body measurements
Indirect calorimetry Cart calorimeter Hand-held calorimeter	Measures resting energy expenditure, respiratory quotient Hand-held calorimeter easy to use and portable, can be used in most clinical settings in patients with cirrhosis Can be used to determine metabolic response to nutrient interventions	Conventional cart-based indirect calorimetry logistically difficult Hand-held calorimetry not as accurate as conventional cart calorimetry

---

Box 1
Factors affecting severity/measures of malnutrition in alcoholic liver disease

- Duration of alcohol use/abuse
- Amount of alcohol consumed
- Time of measurement from last alcohol consumed
- Other underlying causes of liver disease
- Severity of liver disease (Child-Pugh/model for end-stage liver disease score)
- Specific measure used (anthropometry, body composition, circulating proteins, immune function, muscle mass, indirect calorimetry)

---

compelling. Sarcopenia in cirrhosis adversely affects long-term survival,[24] development of other complications of liver disease,[39,40] and post liver transplantation outcomes.[10] Because skeletal muscle is a major nonhepatic organ for ammonia disposal,[41,42] it is intuitively obvious that sarcopenia is accompanied by more severe encephalopathy as was reported recently.[40] Other complications including hospitalizations and infections are also more frequent in malnourished/sarcopenic patients with cirrhosis.[39,40,43] Whether the severity of malnutrition, specifically sarcopenia in ALD, contributes to adverse clinical outcomes is not well studied. Published data that are predominantly descriptive do provide compelling evidence that malnutrition, specifically sarcopenia, is a major adverse consequence of ALD. Interestingly, malnutrition is severe as measured by anthropometric and visceral protein levels in acute alcoholic hepatitis but direct body composition measures and muscle mass by imaging have not been reported.[14,15,34]

Hypermetabolism is another fairly consistent observation in cirrhosis of any cause and contributes to increased mortality.[44] The mechanisms of hypermetabolism and its regulation in cirrhosis are not well understood.[45,46] Whether patients with alcoholic cirrhosis are hypermetabolic to a greater degree than those with nonalcoholic cirrhosis is not known. Interestingly, despite ethanol contributing to "empty calories," patients with alcoholic cirrhosis and alcohol abuse are not obese.[47] This has been suggested to be caused by increased energy expenditure and lower RQ induced by ethanol, which prevents fat accumulation and potentially promotes fat loss.

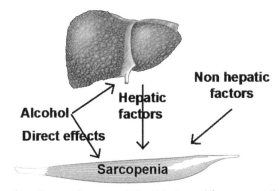

Fig. 1. Schematic of mediators of sarcopenia in ALD. Several factors contribute to sarcopenia in ALD including the direct effects of ethanol or its metabolism in the muscle, ethanol-induced liver disease with consequent hyperammonemia, and nonhepatic factors including gut-derived endotoxemia and cytokine-mediated effects.

Box 2
Factors contributing to sarcopenia in alcoholic liver disease

- Reduced oral intake because of inebriated state
- Anorexia
- Dysguesia
- Low quality of diet
- Hypermetabolism
- Low-sodium diet
- Acute hepatitis-cytokines
- Hyperammonemia of liver disease
- Other complications that affect nutrient intake: gastrointestinal bleeding, encephalopathy
- Diarrhea, portal hypertensive enteropathy with reduced nutrient absorption
- Nausea, emesis

Micronutrient deficiencies have been extensively examined in patients with alcoholism and their replacement should be part of routine clinical practice. Micronutrient deficiencies occur in patients with ALD because the major proportion of calories derived from alcohol lack minerals and vitamins. Specific emphasis is necessary for zinc, vitamin D, thiamine, folate, cyanocobalamin, and selenium.[13] Selenium is gaining interest because of the recognition of selenocysteine and selenoproteins as potential antioxidants in various tissues including skeletal muscle. Whether these mineral deficiencies, including zinc and selenium, contribute to impaired ammonia disposal and protein synthesis is not known.[13,48,49]

In summary, there is clinical recognition of the contribution of malnutrition to poor outcomes but the focus of therapies has always been on reversing the hepatic injury. Lack of effective management strategies for malnutrition in ALD has been mainly caused by the absence of an integrated approach to understand the molecular pathogenesis.[2] An in-depth analysis of the potential molecular mediators of sarcopenia,[50–52] the major component of malnutrition, is beyond the scope of this article but a summary of recent advances is provided next that allows identification of novel therapeutic targets.

MOLECULAR AND METABOLIC PERTURBATIONS CONTRIBUTING TO MALNUTRITION IN ALCOHOLIC LIVER DISEASE

There are two major contributors to sarcopenia in ALD: consequences of liver disease, and the direct effect of ethanol. Liver disease has two major components: hepatic

---

Box 3
Factors specific to alcohol-induced sarcopenia

- Direct metabolism of ethanol by muscle with changes in redox ratio
- Ethanol-induced skeletal muscle mitochondrial dysfunction
- Protein adducts with increased muscle autophagy
- Impaired muscle protein synthesis

---

necroinflammation/fibrosis with hepatocyte dysfunction, and vascular consequences resulting in hepatic bypass of portal circulation. One of the mediators of the liver muscle axis is hyperammonemia, which occurs from impaired hepatic ureagenesis.[42,53–55] The effects of ethanol include lower skeletal muscle protein synthesis,[56–59] increased autophagy,[60] and mitochondrial dysfunction caused by ethanol or its metabolites including acetaldehyde.[61,62] In alcoholic cirrhosis and liver disease, both hyperammonemia and ethanol contribute to muscle loss, which can explain more severe muscle loss in these patients. One of the questions is the relative contribution of ethanol versus hyperammonemia to sarcopenia. Importantly, acetaldehyde, the immediate oxidative product of ethanol, impairs hepatic ureagenesis,[63] the main metabolic disposal pathway for cytotoxic ammonia. This is of immediate clinical and translational relevance because therapeutic targets may be different and the response to therapies may be affected by the impact of these divergent mechanisms. In addition to hyperammonemia and ethanol effects, other alterations including endotoxemia and cytokine alterations in ALD also contribute to sarcopenia by several mechanisms.

Major advances in the understanding of maintenance of skeletal muscle mass and the impact of ethanol on these pathways allows for identifying novel molecular targets **(Fig. 2)**.[50,64] The canonical signaling pathway for protein synthesis is mediated by the Akt/PKB-dependent phosphorylation and activation of target of rapamycin complex

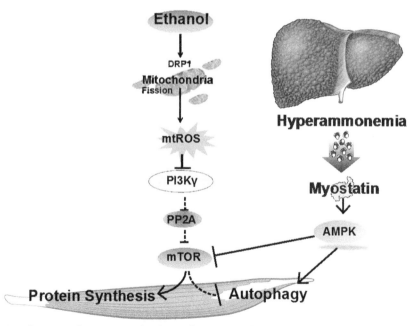

Fig. 2. Schematic of putative molecular pathways contributing to sarcopenia of liver disease. Ethanol or its metabolites (primarily acetaldehyde) activate several pathways either via myostatin or reactive oxygen species–mediated impairment of critical molecular signaling component, mammalian target of rapamycin complex 1 (mTORC1). The consequent reduced protein synthesis and autophagy contribute to sarcopenia and loss of muscle mass. Dephosphorylation of critical regulatory proteins (mTORC1, DRP1) at specific sites causes perturbation of downstream signaling responses. AMPK, AMP kinase; DRP1, dynamin related protein 1 (mitochondrial fission regulatory protein); PI3Kγ, phosphoinositide 3 kinase gamma isoform; PP2A, protein phosphatase 2 A; ROS, reactive oxygen species.

1 (mTORC1), which in turn activates downstream molecules to promote protein synthesis. mTORC1 also inhibits autophagy and ethanol has been reported to inhibit mTORC1 phosphorylation in animal and human studies suggesting that this may be a common mechanism of molecular perturbations and sarcopenia.[60] Interestingly, hyperammonemia also inhibits mTORC1 but the mechanisms may be different. Expression of myostatin, a transforming growth factor-β superfamily member, is increased in response to hyperammonemia and alcohol.[42,59,65] Ethanol activates autophagy via its metabolite acetaldehyde.[60] Skeletal muscle expresses CYP2E1, a component of the microsomal ethanol oxidizing system (MEOS) that metabolizes ethanol and generates reactive oxygen species in addition to mitochondrial dysfunction and mitochondrial reactive oxygen species, targeting either ethanol metabolism or the consequent perturbations may provide novel targets to reverse sarcopenia of ALD.

Several metabolic perturbations also occur in skeletal muscle in response to ethanol exposure. Ethanol is metabolized primarily in the liver, but is also metabolized in nonhepatic (muscle) tissue,[66] where there is increased oxidation via the mitochondrial and nonmitochondrial MEOS. Because MEOS oxidation does not generate much ATP and ethanol causes mitochondrial dysfunction, skeletal muscle ATP content is expected to be lower. Preliminary studies from our laboratory have shown muscle mitochondrial dysfunction and lower ATP content in response to ethanol. Because protein synthesis is one of the most energy-intense processes, it is possible that the additional contribution of impaired ATP synthesis also contributes to sarcopenia. Both molecular perturbations with low mTORC1 activation and low ATP content with increased reactive oxygen species activate autophagy, a protein breakdown mechanism that is additive with the impaired protein synthesis.[42,60] Finally, perturbations caused by ethanol are compounded by ammonia-induced metabolic alterations including lower tricarboxylic acid cycle intermediates in the skeletal muscle that also contribute to reduced muscle mass.

Ethanol induces loss of adipose tissue mass and oxidative stress, and lipolysis, all of which contribute to lower fat mass[47] in addition to reduced muscle mass in patients with ALD.

ROLE OF THE GUT IN MALNUTRITION IN ALCOHOLIC LIVER DISEASE

Gut microbial ammoniagenesis is well recognized and its contribution to hyperammonemia results in not only encephalopathy,[67] but also sarcopenia.[42,68] In addition to the consequences of cirrhosis, ethanol directly impairs absorption, results in defective gut permeability barrier, and alters gut microbiota, all of which contribute to decreased absorption and transport of essential nutrients and endotoxemia.[69–73] There are nascent data that the gut microbiome contributes to skeletal muscle responses but few studies have examined the role of disrupted gut permeability and consequent endotoxemia on nutritional consequences including sarcopenia.[74] Targeting the gut as a potential mechanism to reverse muscle loss and other components of malnutrition including lipopolysaccharide-induced hypermetabolism is a novel area that needs investigation.

MANAGEMENT OF MALNUTRITION IN ALCOHOLIC LIVER DISEASE

The mainstay of the management of malnutrition in ALD has focused on nutrition therapy that has not been effective except in replacing micronutrients (**Box 4**).[18,75] Malnutrition is a broad term and response can depend on the specific component being targeted and the specificity of the measures used to quantify malnutrition. Additionally, treatments that do not target the mechanisms that contribute to malnutrition

---

Box 4
Nutritional supplementation in alcoholic liver disease

Step 1. Abstinence from alcohol

Step 2. Nutritional support: increased protein/calorie intake
　Oral supplementation
　Enteral nutrition
　Parenteral nutrition
　Amino acid supplementation
　Micronutrient replacement

Step 3. Increase physical activity

Step 4. Novel targets
　Myostatin antagonists
　Target of rapamycin complex 1 activators
　Muscle-targeted antioxidants
　Autophagy regulators
　Mitoprotective agents
　Cell-permeable tricarboxylic acid cycle intermediates
　Specific amino acid and analogue supplementation

---

can also explain the lack of effective therapies. Increased protein intake is likely to be of benefit in patients with ALD and those with cirrhosis. However, just providing calories and proteins without altering the translational machinery responsible for peptide chain elongation, decreasing the expression of genes that impair protein synthesis, or altering the mechanisms of protein breakdown via the autophagy pathway contributes to the absence of any definitive measures. Malnutrition and sarcopenia are nearly universal in patients with ALD. Thus, reversing sarcopenia should be an integral therapeutic strategy because this improves survival in cirrhosis.[76] It is, however, not known if improving malnutrition/sarcopenia also improves other outcome measures including encephalopathy, ascites, infection, hospitalizations, and quality of life.

Because cirrhosis is a state of accelerated starvation, strategies to lower RQ may be helpful because low RQ has been correlated with sarcopenia.[28] Late evening snacks, decreasing periods of postprandial or fasting states by providing daytime snacks, preventing prolonged fasting in hospitalized patients for various medical procedures, and encouraging increased protein intake (specifically, low ammoniagenic proteins, such as vegetable proteins) are simple strategies to increase RQ and avoid sarcopenia and its adverse consequences.

Abstinence

Ethanol and its metabolites contribute to malnutrition and sarcopenia by multiple mechanisms. Abstinence should therefore be the mainstay of treating these patients. Continued alcohol use in patients with ALD is likely to result in greater muscle metabolism of ethanol and increased toxicity caused by circulating acetaldehyde generated from the liver. Pharmacotherapy has been of limited success in ensuring abstinence, but a multidisciplinary approach should be part of improving the diet, calorie and protein intake, and reversing sarcopenia.

Nutrition

Several clinical trials and a meta-analysis have been published to date on nutritional support in cirrhosis in general and ALD in particular.[18,20,36,75,77,78] These studies have not been conclusive despite large numbers of patients studied. Reasons for inconclusive results include lack of benefit of oral, enteral, and parenteral supplementation; inconsistency in the measures and definition of nutritional indices and malnutrition; heterogeneous population of patients; variable duration and composition of the supplements; and continued consequences of underlying liver disease and alcohol effects on tissues, primarily the skeletal muscle.

Evaluation of published literature suggests that a daily caloric intake of about 2000 kcal with about 1.2 to 1.5 g/kg/d protein distributed over the day with short intervals between meals to decrease the postabsorptive state is likely to be of benefit in patients with ALD and those with cirrhosis. Different routes of caloric administration can be used.

Oral supplementation may not be effective because of poor intake and compliance from anorexia, dysguesia, impaired absorption, and continued hypermetabolic states. The nonaromatizable anabolic steroid, oxandrolone, showed benefit when added to oral nutritional supplementation.[34,79,80] Late evening snacks with high protein content have the potential to exploit the window of anabolic opportunity at night and prevent muscle loss.[31]

Enteral tube feedings can overcome the effects of anorexia and dysguesia but not poor enteral absorption and have been shown to be beneficial, well-tolerated, and may improve hepatic function but the impact on skeletal muscle and other nutritional parameters is not conclusive.[18]

Parenteral nutrition ensures delivery of nutrients and has been used in patients with ALD. In a comprehensive analysis of parenteral nutrition in ALD, short-term benefits on some nutritional parameters were observed but long-term consequences remain unknown. Parenteral nutrition is associated with significant risks including infections that preclude such supplementation as routine treatment in patients with ALD who have compromised immune function.[18]

Amino acid supplementation including branched-chain amino acids has been used in patients with a variety of liver diseases.[2,13,18,20,77] In acute alcoholic hepatitis there does not seem to be a benefit of branched-chain amino acid supplementation. Meta-analyses of amino acid supplementation for the treatment of cirrhosis and hepatic encephalopathy did not show consistent benefit in nutritional parameters.[2] There may be some benefit in improving visceral protein levels but there are no data on recovery or improvement in skeletal muscle mass in response to amino acid supplementation in patients with cirrhosis with encephalopathy.[81]

Of the essential amino acids, leucine has been investigated the most. In a randomized study in patients with alcoholic cirrhosis, signaling abnormalities in the skeletal muscle and the fractional muscle protein synthesis rate were reversed by a single dose of leucine-enriched branched chain amino acid mixture.[65] These data suggest that much higher doses of leucine may promote skeletal muscle protein synthesis and improve mitochondrial function by increased mitochondrial biogenesis. The use of high-dose leucine or isoleucine in patients with ALD warrants further evaluation.

Exercise in Alcoholic Liver Disease

Increased physical activity improves functional capacity and muscle mass, depending on the type of exercise performed.[82] Alcohol ingestion, either acutely or chronically, impairs exercise capacity, depletes skeletal muscle glycogen stores, and decreases circulating testosterone androgen receptor on the skeletal muscle, all of which impair muscle hypertrophy.[83,84] Exercise also increases muscle ammonia generation that may compound the adverse effects of ethanol.[42,68,85] Muscle strength is decreased because of loss of and impaired function of contractile proteins. There are no data on the response of skeletal muscle to exercise in ALD specifically but data in cirrhosis in general suggests that increasing physical activity improves functional capacity.[82] Whether exercise in addition to nutrient supplementation increases muscle mass in the context of ALD is also not known. Studies on the effects of alcohol on muscle responses to exercise have been conducted only in the context of alcohol ingestion and muscle strength recovers rapidly after stopping alcohol, but it is not known if the hypertrophic responses recover after stopping alcohol.[84,86,87] This is of relevance because ammonia and ethanol potentially complement the adverse effects on molecular signaling pathways in the skeletal muscle[42,60,68] and once abstinence is achieved, persistent hyperammonemia of chronic liver disease may continue to blunt the benefits of exercise. Based on current published data, one may conclude that exercise in combination with abstinence and improved nutrient intake is likely to benefit functional capacity and muscle mass in ALD.

NOVEL THERAPEUTIC TARGETS
Myostatin

The initial report in rats that ethanol feeding increased myostatin expression that was reversed by administration of insulin-like growth factor 1 as a binary complex[59] was followed by a report that myostatin expression was increased in alcoholic cirrhosis.[65] Several strategies to block myostatin including monoclonal antibodies, follistatin, and antagomirs have the potential to reverse muscle loss in ALD.[50]

Muscle-Targeted Antioxidants

Mitochondrial and nonmitochondrial sites of reactive oxygen species with oxidative stress occur in the skeletal muscle. Mitochondrial-targeted catalase, mitochondrial fission inhibitor, and p110 are novel agents that may be helpful.[88] In prior studies, antioxidant supplementation has generally not been therapeutically effective.[48,89] However, novel methods to target specific sites of reactive oxygen species generation may be beneficial and warrant investigation.

Autophagy Regulators

Because increased skeletal muscle autophagy contributes to muscle loss, pharmacologic regulators of autophagy may be a potential treatment option. Both inhibitors and activators of autophagy have been developed and can be used to modulate autophagy. Another option is to identify the mechanism by which ethanol activates autophagy and controls the initiation of dysregulated autophagy.

Mitoprotective Agents

Mitochondrial fission and fragmentation occur in response to cellular stress and ethanol exposure in mice, and targeting mitochondrial fission machinery is a potential therapeutic approach.[88] Ethanol also causes a reduction in tricarboxylic acid cycle intermediates and providing cell permeable esters of these intermediates holds promise not only to provide anaplerotic substrates but also a novel method to remove ammonia by conversion to glutamine.

SUMMARY

The lack of common data elements/standardized definitions of various terms that are included under the term "malnutrition" has resulted in difficulty in interpreting data from different groups. Because sarcopenia is the major component of "malnutrition," future studies evaluating interventions should include sarcopenia as an outcome measure. Because muscle mass changes slowly over time, other more acute measures are needed including changes in resting energy expenditure and RQ using the easily accessible hand-held calorimeters. Increasing calories and high-quality proteins alone are clearly insufficient and targeting molecular and metabolic perturbations is likely a more successful strategy. The anticipated increase in proportion and number of patients with ALD in the next decades, limited therapeutic armamentarium to treat alcohol use, and continued organ shortage for transplantation make it imperative to develop novel and effective nontransplant treatments for ALD. Improving muscle mass is expected to increase survival, improve quality of life, and lower the incidence of other complications in patients and should form a priority area for future clinical studies in patients with ALD.

REFERENCES

1. Periyalwar P, Dasarathy S. Malnutrition in cirrhosis: contribution and consequences of sarcopenia on metabolic and clinical responses. Clin Liver Dis 2012;16(1):95–131.
2. Dasarathy S. Consilience in sarcopenia of cirrhosis. J Cachexia Sarcopenia Muscle 2012;3(4):225–37.
3. Common Data Elements Portal at NIH. Available at: https://www.nlm.nih.gov/cde/. Accessed December 20, 2015.
4. Merli M, Romiti A, Riggio O, et al. Optimal nutritional indexes in chronic liver disease. JPEN J Parenter Enteral Nutr 1987;11(Suppl 5):130S–4S.
5. Romiti A, Merli M, Martorano M, et al. Malabsorption and nutritional abnormalities in patients with liver cirrhosis. Ital J Gastroenterol 1990;22(3):118–23.
6. Alberino F, Gatta A, Amodio P, et al. Nutrition and survival in patients with liver cirrhosis. Nutrition 2001;17(6):445–50.
7. Brown LA, Cook RT, Jerrells TR, et al. Acute and chronic alcohol abuse modulate immunity. Alcohol Clin Exp Res 2006;30(9):1624–31.
8. Klipstein-Grobusch K, Georg T, Boeing H. Interviewer variability in anthropometric measurements and estimates of body composition. Int J Epidemiol 1997;26(Suppl 1):S174–80.
9. Rosenberg IH. Sarcopenia: origins and clinical relevance. J Nutr 1997;127(Suppl 5):990S–1S.
10. Englesbe MJ, Patel SP, He K, et al. Sarcopenia and mortality after liver transplantation. J Am Coll Surg 2010;211(2):271–8.
11. Dasarathy S, McCullough AJ, Muc S, et al. Sarcopenia associated with portosystemic shunting is reversed by follistatin. J Hepatol 2011;54(5):915–21.
12. Mohammad MK, Zhou Z, Cave M, et al. Zinc and liver disease. Nutr Clin Pract 2012;27(1):8–20.
13. Leevy CM, Moroianu SA. Nutritional aspects of alcoholic liver disease. Clin Liver Dis 2005;9(1):67–81.
14. Mendenhall CL, Moritz TE, Roselle GA, et al. A study of oral nutritional support with oxandrolone in malnourished patients with alcoholic hepatitis: results of a Department of Veterans Affairs cooperative study. Hepatology 1993;17(4):564–76.
15. Mendenhall CL, Moritz TE, Roselle GA, et al. Protein energy malnutrition in severe alcoholic hepatitis: diagnosis and response to treatment. The VA Cooperative Study Group #275. JPEN J Parenter Enteral Nutr 1995;19(4):258–65.

16. Gonzalez-Reimers E, Fernandez-Rodriguez CM, Santolaria-Fernandez F, et al. Interleukin-15 and other myokines in chronic alcoholics. Alcohol Alcohol 2011; 46(5):529–33.
17. Pedersen BK. Muscles and their myokines. J Exp Biol 2011;214(Pt 2):337–46.
18. Halsted CH. Nutrition and alcoholic liver disease. Semin Liver Dis 2004;24(3): 289–304.
19. Mullen KD, Dasarathy S. Potential new therapies for alcoholic liver disease. Clin Liver Dis 1988;2(4):851–81.
20. Stickel F, Hoehn B, Schuppan D, et al. Review article: nutritional therapy in alcoholic liver disease. Aliment Pharmacol Ther 2003;18(4):357–73.
21. Guglielmi FW, Panella C, Buda A, et al. Nutritional state and energy balance in cirrhotic patients with or without hypermetabolism. Multicentre prospective study by the 'Nutritional Problems in Gastroenterology' Section of the Italian Society of Gastroenterology (SIGE). Dig Liver Dis 2005;37(9):681–8.
22. Campillo B, Richardet JP, Scherman E, et al. Evaluation of nutritional practice in hospitalized cirrhotic patients: results of a prospective study. Nutrition 2003; 19(6):515–21.
23. Guirguis J, Chhatwal J, Dasarathy J, et al. Clinical impact of alcohol-related cirrhosis in the next decade: estimates based on current epidemiological trends in the United States. Alcohol Clin Exp Res 2015;39(11):2085–94.
24. Montano-Loza AJ, Meza-Junco J, Prado CM, et al. Muscle wasting is associated with mortality in patients with cirrhosis. Clin Gastroenterol Hepatol 2012;10(2): 166–73, 173.e1.
25. Dasarathy J, Alkhouri N, Dasarathy S. Changes in body composition after transjugular intrahepatic portosystemic stent in cirrhosis: a critical review of literature. Liver Int 2011;31(9):1250–8.
26. Shen W, Punyanitya M, Wang Z, et al. Total body skeletal muscle and adipose tissue volumes: estimation from a single abdominal cross-sectional image. J Appl Physiol (1985) 2004;97(6):2333–8.
27. Bemben MG. Use of diagnostic ultrasound for assessing muscle size. J Strength Cond Res 2002;16(1):103–8.
28. Glass C, Hipskind P, Tsien C, et al. Sarcopenia and a physiologically low respiratory quotient in patients with cirrhosis: a prospective controlled study. J Appl Physiol (1985) 2013;114(5):559–65.
29. Tsien C, Garber A, Narayanan A, et al. Post-liver transplantation sarcopenia in cirrhosis: a prospective evaluation. J Gastroenterol Hepatol 2014;29(6):1250–7.
30. Plank LD, Gane EJ, Peng S, et al. Nocturnal nutritional supplementation improves total body protein status of patients with liver cirrhosis: a randomized 12-month trial. Hepatology 2008;48(2):557–66.
31. Tsien CD, McCullough AJ, Dasarathy S. Late evening snack: exploiting a period of anabolic opportunity in cirrhosis. J Gastroenterol Hepatol 2012;27(3):430–41.
32. Hipskind P, Glass C, Charlton D, et al. Do handheld calorimeters have a role in assessment of nutrition needs in hospitalized patients? A systematic review of literature. Nutr Clin Pract 2011;26(4):426–33.
33. Glass C, Hipskind P, Cole D, et al. Handheld calorimeter is a valid instrument to quantify resting energy expenditure in hospitalized cirrhotic patients: a prospective study. Nutr Clin Pract 2012;27(5):677–88.
34. Mendenhall C, Roselle GA, Gartside P, et al. Relationship of protein calorie malnutrition to alcoholic liver disease: a reexamination of data from two Veterans Administration Cooperative Studies. Alcohol Clin Exp Res 1995;19(3):635–41.

35. Caregaro L, Alberino F, Amodio P, et al. Malnutrition in alcoholic and virus-related cirrhosis. Am J Clin Nutr 1996;63(4):602–9.

36. McClain CJ, Barve SS, Barve A, et al. Alcoholic liver disease and malnutrition. Alcohol Clin Exp Res 2011;35(5):815–20.

37. Hanai T, Shiraki M, Nishimura K, et al. Sarcopenia impairs prognosis of patients with liver cirrhosis. Nutrition 2015;31(1):193–9.

38. Huisman EJ, Trip EJ, Siersema PD, et al. Protein energy malnutrition predicts complications in liver cirrhosis. Eur J Gastroenterol Hepatol 2011;23(11):982–9.

39. Merli M, Nicolini G, Angeloni S, et al. Malnutrition is a risk factor in cirrhotic patients undergoing surgery. Nutrition 2002;18(11–12):978–86.

40. Merli M, Giusto M, Lucidi C, et al. Muscle depletion increases the risk of overt and minimal hepatic encephalopathy: results of a prospective study. Metab Brain Dis 2013;28(2):281–4.

41. Lockwood AH, McDonald JM, Reiman RE, et al. The dynamics of ammonia metabolism in man. Effects of liver disease and hyperammonemia. J Clin Invest 1979; 63(3):449–60.

42. Qiu J, Thapaliya S, Runkana A, et al. Hyperammonemia in cirrhosis induces transcriptional regulation of myostatin by an NF-kappaB-mediated mechanism. Proc Natl Acad Sci U S A 2013;110(45):18162–7.

43. Merli M, Lucidi C, Giannelli V, et al. Cirrhotic patients are at risk for health care-associated bacterial infections. Clin Gastroenterol Hepatol 2010;8(11):979–85.

44. Peng S, Plank LD, McCall JL, et al. Body composition, muscle function, and energy expenditure in patients with liver cirrhosis: a comprehensive study. Am J Clin Nutr 2007;85(5):1257–66.

45. Muller MJ, Bottcher J, Selberg O, et al. Hypermetabolism in clinically stable patients with liver cirrhosis. Am J Clin Nutr 1999;69(6):1194–201.

46. Mathur S, Peng S, Gane EJ, et al. Hypermetabolism predicts reduced transplant-free survival independent of MELD and Child-Pugh scores in liver cirrhosis. Nutrition 2007;23(5):398–403.

47. Levine JA, Harris MM, Morgan MY. Energy expenditure in chronic alcohol abuse. Eur J Clin Invest 2000;30(9):779–86.

48. Ward RJ, Peters TJ. The antioxidant status of patients with either alcohol-induced liver damage or myopathy. Alcohol Alcohol 1992;27(4):359–65.

49. Rua RM, Ojeda ML, Nogales F, et al. Serum selenium levels and oxidative balance as differential markers in hepatic damage caused by alcohol. Life Sci 2014;94(2):158–63.

50. Cohen S, Nathan JA, Goldberg AL. Muscle wasting in disease: molecular mechanisms and promising therapies. Nat Rev Drug Discov 2015;14(1):58–74.

51. Lang CH, Frost RA, Summer AD, et al. Molecular mechanisms responsible for alcohol-induced myopathy in skeletal muscle and heart. Int J Biochem Cell Biol 2005;37(10):2180–95.

52. Fernandez-Sola J, Preedy VR, Lang CH, et al. Molecular and cellular events in alcohol-induced muscle disease. Alcohol Clin Exp Res 2007;31(12):1953–62.

53. Rudman D, DiFulco TJ, Galambos JT, et al. Maximal rates of excretion and synthesis of urea in normal and cirrhotic subjects. J Clin Invest 1973;52(9):2241–9.

54. Nomura F, Ohnishi K, Terabayashi H, et al. Effect of intrahepatic portal-systemic shunting on hepatic ammonia extraction in patients with cirrhosis. Hepatology 1994;20(6):1478–81.

55. Shangraw RE, Jahoor F. Effect of liver disease and transplantation on urea synthesis in humans: relationship to acid-base status. Am J Physiol 1999; 276(5 Pt 1):G1145–52.

56. Steiner JL, Lang CH. Alcohol impairs skeletal muscle protein synthesis and mTOR signaling in a time-dependent manner following electrically stimulated muscle contraction. J Appl Physiol (1985) 2014;117(10):1170–9.
57. Kumar V, Frost RA, Lang CH. Alcohol impairs insulin and IGF-I stimulation of S6K1 but not 4E-BP1 in skeletal muscle. Am J Physiol Endocrinol Metab 2002;283(5):E917–28.
58. Lang CH, Pruznak AM, Deshpande N, et al. Alcohol intoxication impairs phosphorylation of S6K1 and S6 in skeletal muscle independently of ethanol metabolism. Alcohol Clin Exp Res 2004;28(11):1758–67.
59. Lang CH, Frost RA, Svanberg E, et al. IGF-I/IGFBP-3 ameliorates alterations in protein synthesis, eIF4E availability, and myostatin in alcohol-fed rats. Am J Physiol Endocrinol Metab 2004;286(6):E916–26.
60. Thapaliya S, Runkana A, McMullen MR, et al. Alcohol-induced autophagy contributes to loss in skeletal muscle mass. Autophagy 2014;10(4):677–90.
61. Lang CH, Lynch CJ, Vary TC. Alcohol-induced IGF-I resistance is ameliorated in mice deficient for mitochondrial branched-chain aminotransferase. J Nutr 2010;140(5):932–8.
62. Mansouri A, Demeilliers C, Amsellem S, et al. Acute ethanol administration oxidatively damages and depletes mitochondrial DNA in mouse liver, brain, heart, and skeletal muscles: protective effects of antioxidants. J Pharmacol Exp Ther 2001;298(2):737–43.
63. Holmuhamedov EL, Czerny C, Beeson CC, et al. Ethanol suppresses ureagenesis in rat hepatocytes: role of acetaldehyde. J Biol Chem 2012;287(10):7692–700.
64. Steiner JL, Lang CH. Dysregulation of skeletal muscle protein metabolism by alcohol. Am J Physiol Endocrinol Metab 2015;308(9):E699–712.
65. Tsien C, Davuluri G, Singh D, et al. Metabolic and molecular responses to leucine-enriched branched chain amino acid supplementation in the skeletal muscle of alcoholic cirrhosis. Hepatology 2015;61(6):2018–29.
66. Dam G, Sorensen M, Munk OL, et al. Hepatic ethanol elimination kinetics in patients with cirrhosis. Scand J Gastroenterol 2009;44(7):867–71.
67. Dasarathy S. Role of gut bacteria in the therapy of hepatic encephalopathy with lactulose and antibiotics. Indian J Gastroenterol 2003;22(Suppl 2):S50–3.
68. Qiu J, Tsien C, Thapalaya S, et al. Hyperammonemia-mediated autophagy in skeletal muscle contributes to sarcopenia of cirrhosis. Am J Physiol Endocrinol Metab 2012;303(8):E983–93.
69. World MJ, Ryle PR, Thomson AD. Alcoholic malnutrition and the small intestine. Alcohol Alcohol 1985;20(2):89–124.
70. Chaudhry KK, Shukla PK, Mir H, et al. Glutamine supplementation attenuates ethanol-induced disruption of apical junctional complexes in colonic epithelium and ameliorates gut barrier dysfunction and fatty liver in mice. J Nutr Biochem 2016;27:16–26.
71. Zhong W, Li Q, Sun Q, et al. Preventing gut leakiness and endotoxemia contributes to the protective effect of zinc on alcohol-induced steatohepatitis in rats. J Nutr 2015;145(12):2690–8.
72. Forsyth CB, Tang Y, Shaikh M, et al. Role of snail activation in alcohol-induced iNOS-mediated disruption of intestinal epithelial cell permeability. Alcohol Clin Exp Res 2011;35(9):1635–43.
73. Bala S, Marcos M, Gattu A, et al. Acute binge drinking increases serum endotoxin and bacterial DNA levels in healthy individuals. PLoS One 2014;9(5):e96864.
74. Norman K, Pirlich M, Schulzke JD, et al. Increased intestinal permeability in malnourished patients with liver cirrhosis. Eur J Clin Nutr 2012;66(10):1116–9.

75. Antar R, Wong P, Ghali P. A meta-analysis of nutritional supplementation for management of hospitalized alcoholic hepatitis. Can J Gastroenterol 2012; 26(7):463–7.
76. Tsien C, Shah SN, McCullough AJ, et al. Reversal of sarcopenia predicts survival after a transjugular intrahepatic portosystemic stent. Eur J Gastroenterol Hepatol 2013;25(1):85–93.
77. Nasrallah SM, Galambos JT. Aminoacid therapy of alcoholic hepatitis. Lancet 1980;2(8207):1276–7.
78. Calvey H, Davis M, Williams R. Controlled trial of nutritional supplementation, with and without branched chain amino acid enrichment, in treatment of acute alcoholic hepatitis. J Hepatol 1985;1(2):141–51.
79. Bonkovsky HL, Singh RH, Jafri IH, et al. A randomized, controlled trial of treatment of alcoholic hepatitis with parenteral nutrition and oxandrolone. II. Short-term effects on nitrogen metabolism, metabolic balance, and nutrition. Am J Gastroenterol 1991;86(9):1209–18.
80. Orr R, Fiatarone Singh M. The anabolic androgenic steroid oxandrolone in the treatment of wasting and catabolic disorders: review of efficacy and safety. Drugs 2004;64(7):725–50.
81. Olde Damink SW, Jalan R, Deutz NE, et al. Isoleucine infusion during "simulated" upper gastrointestinal bleeding improves liver and muscle protein synthesis in cirrhotic patients. Hepatology 2007;45(3):560–8.
82. Jones JC, Coombes JS, Macdonald GA. Exercise capacity and muscle strength in patients with cirrhosis. Liver Transpl 2012;18(2):146–51.
83. Peters TJ, Nikolovski S, Raja GK, et al. Ethanol acutely impairs glycogen repletion in skeletal muscle following high intensity short duration exercise in the rat. Addict Biol 1996;1(3):289–95.
84. Vingren JL, Koziris LP, Gordon SE, et al. Chronic alcohol intake, resistance training, and muscle androgen receptor content. Med Sci Sports Exerc 2005; 37(11):1842–8.
85. Graham TE, Turcotte LP, Kiens B, et al. Effect of endurance training on ammonia and amino acid metabolism in humans. Med Sci Sports Exerc 1997;29(5): 646–53.
86. Barnes MJ, Mundel T, Stannard SR. A low dose of alcohol does not impact skeletal muscle performance after exercise-induced muscle damage. Eur J Appl Physiol 2011;111(4):725–9.
87. Haugvad A, Haugvad L, Hamarsland H, et al. Ethanol does not delay muscle recovery but decreases testosterone/cortisol ratio. Med Sci Sports Exerc 2014; 46(11):2175–83.
88. Qi X, Qvit N, Su YC, et al. A novel Drp1 inhibitor diminishes aberrant mitochondrial fission and neurotoxicity. J Cell Sci 2013;126(Pt 3):789–802.
89. Fernandez-Sola J, Villegas E, Nicolas JM, et al. Serum and muscle levels of alpha-tocopherol, ascorbic acid, and retinol are normal in chronic alcoholic myopathy. Alcohol Clin Exp Res 1998;22(2):422–7.

Long-Term Management of Alcoholic Liver Disease

Sanath Allampati, MD[a],*, Kevin D. Mullen, MD[b]

KEYWORDS

- Alcoholic liver disease • Varices • Abstinence • Recidivism
- Hepatocellular carcinoma

KEY POINTS

- The absolute key to the management of alcoholic liver disease is early recognition by the patient and the physician.
- Excessive alcohol consumption, ranging from drinking more than recommended amounts to abuse, is one of the most preventable causes of death and disability.
- The US Preventive Services Task Force guidelines recommend screening for alcoholism in the primary care setting.
- Abstinence is the cornerstone of therapy and it decreases mortality and morbidity significantly.
- Alcoholic cirrhosis can cause varices that need to be followed closely with upper endoscopy to prevent or treat hemorrhage.

INTRODUCTION

Most established gastroenterology practices in the United States that deal with liver disease look after many patients with alcoholic liver disease (ALD), with the data that approximately two-thirds of Americans drink some amount of alcohol.[1] The absolute key to the management of ALD is early recognition by the patient and the physician that excessive daily alcohol intake is occurring (>60 g/d).[2] It is striking how often patients will virtually deny significant alcohol intake until repeated questioning gets them to reveal the problem. Overly aggressive approaches to patients with probable overconsumption of alcohol can, however, be counterproductive. Indeed, the patient may leave the practice altogether. In any event, it can take a number of visits to identify heavy alcohol consumption. Many physicians do not really probe the situation critically and later discover severe alcohol abuse problems. Clearly, the sooner the alcohol

The authors have nothing to disclose.
[a] Department of Clinical Nutrition, Cleveland Clinic Foundation, 9500 Euclid Avenue, Cleveland, OH 44195, USA; [b] MetroHealth Medical Center, Cleveland, OH 44195, USA
* Corresponding author.
E-mail address: sanathallampati@gmail.com

Clin Liver Dis 20 (2016) 551–562
http://dx.doi.org/10.1016/j.cld.2016.02.011
1089-3261/16/$ – see front matter © 2016 Elsevier Inc. All rights reserved.

liver.theclinics.com

consumption problem is identified, the better the chances are to avoid developing ALD and subsequent cirrhosis. In this review, we describe an approach to long-term management of ALD that is outlined in the algorithm in **Fig. 1**.

MANAGEMENT OF ALCOHOLISM
Screening for Problem Drinking

Excessive alcohol consumption, ranging from drinking more than recommended amounts to abuse, is one of the most preventable causes of death and disability.[3] Patients who drink more than 60 g/d are at risk for alcohol-related health problems. The US Preventive Services Task Force (USPSTF) guidelines recommend screening for alcoholism in the primary care setting.[4] This is aimed at detecting and treating alcohol abuse at an early stage before significant liver disease has occurred.

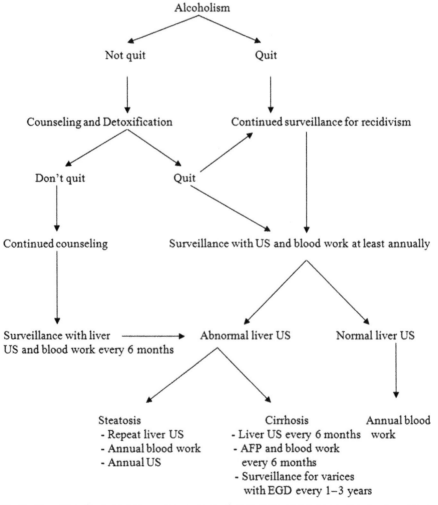

Fig. 1. Algorithm for long-term management of ALD. EGD, esophagogastroduodenoscopy; US, ultrasound.

Direct questioning is the most practical way to establish if a patient has excessive alcohol intake. A number of tools/questionnaires have been developed to formally screen for problem drinking (**Box 1**). The CAGE questionnaire is a validated screening questionnaire for alcohol use disorders.[5] The Alcohol Use Disorders Identification Test (AUDIT) questionnaire is recommended by the World Health Organization, National Institute of Alcohol Abuse and Alcoholism, and USPSTF to screen for alcohol abuse in primary care. AUDIT-C, which is a shorter version, is widely validated and is effective in identifying hazardous drinkers or those with active alcohol use disorder. The Short Michigan Alcohol Screening Test (SMAST) questionnaire is used for diagnosing alcoholism in primary care and SMAST-G is effective in identifying hazardous drinkers in elderly men.[6] In addition, the determination of lifetime alcohol consumption with the help of a structured interview and instruments like Lifetime Drinking History is very important.[7]

Abstinence Therapies

Alcohol abstinence is the key to the long-term treatment of patients with ALD. Pharmacotherapy has emerged as an important tool in the treatment of alcohol abuse and the alcohol withdrawal syndrome. Several medications have been tried but only a few of them have shown successful results in terms of achieving abstinence from alcohol (**Box 2**). Disulfiram inhibits aldehyde dehydrogenase, which leads to accumulation of acetaldehyde.[8] This accumulation of acetaldehyde causes aversion to further alcohol use and is indicated for prevention of relapse in abstinent patients. Significant hepatotoxicity has curtailed its use in controlling alcohol intake. Naltrexone and nalmefene, μ-opioid antagonists, decrease the rewarding effects of alcohol and consequently reduce intake and cravings for alcohol.[9] Acamprosate diminishes the craving for alcohol by reinstating the balance between excitatory and inhibitory neurotransmitters.[10] Gamma-hydroxy butyrate (GHB) has been approved in parts of Europe and its mechanism of action has been that of substitution therapy.[11] The benefits

---

Box 1
Alcohol questionnaires used for screening of alcohol consumption/screening tools for alcohol abuse

1. CAGE questionnaire: 4-part questionnaire
   a. Validated screening technique for identifying alcoholism
   b. Detects 93% of excessive drinkers

2. AUDIT questionnaire: Alcohol Use Disorders Identification Test
   a. 10-question test
   b. Effective in detecting alcohol use disorder in men
   c. Most effective in identifying problem drinking among elderly men

3. AUDIT-C questionnaire: 3-question screening test
   a. Identifies hazardous drinkers or those with active alcohol use disorder

4. SMAST: Short Michigan Alcohol Screening Test
   a. 13-question test
   b. Used for diagnosing alcoholism within primary care
   c. Not recommended for screening purposes

5. SMAST-G: geriatric version
   a. 10-question test
   b. More focused on geriatric patients
   c. Effective in identifying hazardous drinking in elderly men

---

Box 2
Medical treatments to reduce alcohol intake

- Disulfiram (approved in Europe and by the Food and Drug Administration [FDA])
- Naltrexone (approved in Europe and by FDA)
- Acamprosate (approved in Europe and by FDA)
- Nalmefene (approved in Europe)
- Benzodiazepines
  ○ Diazepam
  ○ Chlordiazepoxide
  ○ Lorazepam
- Gamma-hydroxy butyrate (GHB)
- Baclofen
- Topiramate
- Buspirone
- Varenicline
- Anticonvulsants
  ○ Carbamazepine
  ○ Valproic acid
  ○ Phenytoin
- Combination of naltrexone and acamprosate
- Combination of ondansetron and naltrexone

Medications being tested in trials

- Pregabalin
- Gabapentin
- Prazosin
- Ondansetron

---

derived from the current medical therapies are modest and more effective medications are needed. Medications currently being studied for future use in the management of alcoholism are also included in **Box 2**.

Recidivism

An important aspect of alcoholism is the tendency for recidivism, resumption of alcohol use, often heavy, after periods of abstinence. One of the major reasons to have regular office visits is to try to detect relapse of alcoholism. Indeed, one can argue that regular office visits every 6 months are crucial for the management of patients with ALD. This is primarily because of the dual goal of stopping alcohol consumption and detecting the development of structural liver disease. If the patient relapses, he or she needs to be assessed by detoxification and chemical dependency experts. Referring patients to detoxification clinics is usually not successful if the patient has no desire to stop consuming alcohol (see **Fig. 1**).

Natural History of Alcoholic Liver Disease

The following sections of this review outline the management of ALD before and after cirrhosis becomes established. Generally, 90% of patients consuming more than 60 g/d of alcohol will have fatty liver.[12] Total abstinence from alcohol can result in clearance of all fat in 1 to 2 months. Interestingly, 5% to 15% of these total abstainers will still go on to progress to alcoholic hepatitis and ultimately cirrhosis.[13] It has been emphasized that all 3 features of ALD (steatosis, alcoholic hepatitis, and cirrhosis) can be seen in liver biopsy alongside each other in some patients.[14] If, after alcohol cessation for some time, the patient resumes heavy alcohol intake, there is a threefold increase in the tendency to develop severe fibrosis and or cirrhosis.

Before cirrhosis becomes established, patients with ALD can suffer from the collection of other disorders that are a consequence of long-term alcohol abuse, as outlined in **Box 3**.

DIAGNOSIS OF ALCOHOLIC LIVER DISEASE
Clinical and Laboratory Findings

The history and physical is still important in helping raise suspicion that underlying ALD is present. We find spider angiomata to be particularly helpful in suggesting cirrhosis, especially in male patients. Other stigmata of chronic liver disease, such as ascites, or gynecomastia when coupled with history of alcoholism can be helpful in diagnosing alcoholic cirrhosis. However, laboratory testing needs to be done to rule out other causes of chronic liver disease, including viral hepatitis, hemochromatosis, and other hereditary liver disorders. Thrombocytopenia can be helpful in indicating underlying cirrhosis. However, direct effects of alcohol on bone marrow production may also induce thrombocytopenia.

Laboratory testing is somewhat helpful in identifying the presence of ALD. Most patients with just fatty liver will have either normal transaminases or modestly elevated aspartate transaminase (AST) and alanine transaminase (ALT) levels. Typically, the transaminases are less than 200 IU/L with AST being 2 to 4 times higher than the ALT level. When alcoholic hepatitis (AH) occurs, bilirubin elevations are common, and the bilirubin level is a prognostic sign for the severity of AH. Even though AH is a more advanced consequence of ALD, the transaminases are still elevated only threefold to fivefold over normal with an AST/ALT index greater than 2. Alcoholic

---

Box 3
Toxic effects of excessive alcohol consumption
Wernicke-Korsakoff syndrome
Macrocytic anemia
Thrombocytopenia
Cancer of mouth, trachea, esophagus, liver, breast, and colorectal region
Cardiomyopathy
Dementia
Depression
Seizures
Gout
Hypertension
Pancreatitis
Increased risk of diabetes mellitus type 2

foamy degeneration, a variant of AH, is associated with much higher transaminases (500 IU/L) than in standard AH.[15]

Because of the relative frequency of ALD with multiple other causes of liver disease, such as hepatitis B and C, as well as drug hepatotoxicity (especially acetaminophen), the pattern of liver test abnormalities usually seen in ALD may be altered considerably.

Imaging

One of the major roles of imaging in ALD is to rule out other causes of liver disease, especially obstructive biliary pathology or infiltrative and neoplastic diseases of the liver.[16] MRI can be helpful in distinguishing end-stage liver disease related to viral hepatitis infection from ALD. All 3 imaging techniques are capable of detecting nodularity of the liver in cirrhosis and are essential in identifying select areas for biopsy to rule out hepatocellular carcinoma (HCC). This is discussed later in the section on screening for HCC.

Role of Liver Biopsy in Alcoholic Liver Disease

The role of liver biopsy in ALD these days, primarily, is to ensure that no other liver disease is present in the patient. It has been noted that histologic confirmation of AH is present in only 70% to 80% of patients when a liver biopsy is performed.[17] This raises the issue of the accuracy of clinicians in diagnosing ALD without a liver biopsy. Liver biopsy in a patient with coagulopathy from advanced liver disease is a challenge that can be circumvented by the use of transjugular liver biopsy. In our practice, we are very selective in performing liver biopsies in patients with ALD. We tend to biopsy primarily to look for evidence of other liver diseases.

Management of Alcoholic Liver Disease

Abstinence is the cornerstone of therapy and it decreases mortality and morbidity significantly. Five-year mortality decreases from 30% to 10% in people who abstain from alcohol when compared with those who continue to drink.[18] Continued alcohol consumption increases portal pressures and increases porto-collateral blood flow in cirrhotic patients and significantly worsens hepatic hemodynamics. This leads to an increase in variceal bleeding episodes. In addition, abstinence decreases hepatic fibrosis and rate of rebleeding after acute variceal hemorrhage. More importantly, most transplant programs require prolonged periods of abstinence before the patients can become eligible for liver transplantation.

In addition to continued drinking, nutritional deficiencies are associated with increased morbidity and mortality. Weight loss, muscle wasting, and nutritional deficiencies are commonly noted in patients with ALD, and they could result from poor dietary intake from anorexia, altered sense of taste and smell, nausea and vomiting, impaired absorption, and impaired protein synthesis from cytokine-induced inflammatory responses.[19] The commonly encountered nutritional deficiencies are fat-soluble vitamins, B vitamins like thiamine, folate, niacin, pyridoxine, and trace elements.[20] It is suggested that support in the form of enteral or parenteral nutrition improves survival and also decreases complications after liver transplantation in patients with ALD. Regular assessment for nutritional deficiencies and supplementation as needed (**Box 4**) and a high-protein diet with frequent interval feedings focusing on breakfast and nighttime snack are strongly recommended with the aim of decreasing wasting in patients with ALD and cirrhosis.[21]

Multiple medical treatments have also been suggested for long-term treatment of ALD (see **Box 4**), but more studies are needed to prove that these treatments improve morbidity and mortality in patients with ALD.

Box 4
Nutrition and medical treatment of alcoholic liver disease

1. Nutritional support: all patients with alcoholic liver disease (ALD) should be assessed for nutritional deficiencies, both protein-calorie and vitamin and mineral.
   a. Supplementation with dietary branched chain amino acids improves encephalopathy, nitrogen balance, and serum bilirubin
   b. Supplemental protein decreases hospitalizations for infections in decompensated patients
   c. Multiple feedings, emphasizing breakfast and a nighttime snack with a regular oral diet at higher than usual dietary intake (1.2–1.5 g/kg for protein and 35–40 kcal/kg for energy)

2. Propylthiouracil: decreased risk of mortality in ALD
   a. Serious side effects extremely rare
   b. Not recommended at this time; more trials needed

3. Colchicine: decreased long-term mortality rate of patients with alcoholic cirrhosis
   a. May decrease risk of cirrhosis
   b. Not recommended at this time; more trials needed

4. S-adenosyl methionine: decreased mortality and liver transplantation in patients with alcoholic cirrhosis
   a. Increased survival in patients with alcoholic cirrhosis
   b. Only recommended for clinical trials

5. Silymarin: increased survival in patients with alcoholic cirrhosis.
   a. Not recommended at this time

Alcoholic Liver Disease Without Cirrhosis

The presence of cirrhosis is not always easy to establish. Thus, clinical judgment must be used to decide on surveillance programs. Depending on the clinical circumstances, the surveillance testing may need to be done more frequently to overcome the inaccuracy in diagnosing cirrhosis. Liver biopsy is subject to sampling error, so complete reliance on liver biopsy cannot be recommended to identify all patients have cirrhosis and are at risk of developing HCC. Generally, the risk of HCC is greatly increased in patients with cirrhosis. However, even in patients with lesser stage of liver fibrosis, there is still a risk for developing HCC. Therefore, some physicians recommend annual liver imaging for all patients with ALD, even those without cirrhosis. It is our recommendation that all patients with or without cirrhosis be seen every 6 months to monitor for recidivism and further deterioration of liver disease.

Alcoholic Liver Disease with Cirrhosis

Multiple long-term complications can occur in patients with alcoholic cirrhosis. These include gastroesophageal varices, HCC, hepatic encephalopathy, ascites, hepatorenal syndrome, and hepatic hydrothorax. This section focuses on gastroesophageal varices and HCC.

Gastroesophageal varices

Cirrhosis, from any etiology, can lead to portal hypertension. Initially, resistance to blood flow through the liver is encountered due to developing fibrosis and regenerative nodules in the liver.[22,23] This is compounded by the intrahepatic vasoconstriction due to diminished endogenous nitric oxide production.[24] There is also a component of increased blood flow through the portal vein resulting from splanchnic arteriolar vasodilatation.[25] These hemodynamic changes lead to bypass of the liver by blood that takes the route of lesser resistance with the resultant formation of gastroesophageal varices. They are noted in approximately 50% of patients with cirrhosis including 40% of Child-Pugh class A patients and 85% of Child-Pugh class C patients.[26] Patients with cirrhosis who do not have varices at the time of presentation develop them at a rate of 8% per year.[27] Hepatic venous pressure gradient (HVPG) of greater than 10 mm Hg is a strong predictor for development of varices in patients with cirrhosis who do not have them at the time of presentation.[28] When the HVPG is reduced to less than 12 mm Hg, the risk of variceal hemorrhage is significantly diminished.[29]

The gold standard test to diagnose varices is esophagogastroduodenoscopy (EGD). An EGD should be performed in every patient when diagnosed with cirrhosis.[30] In patients with compensated cirrhosis with no varices on initial EGD, repeat EGD should be performed in 2 to 3 years.[22] When small varices are seen at presentation, EGD should be repeated in 1 to 2 years.[22] In patients with decompensated cirrhosis, EGD should be done on an annual basis regardless of the size of the varices.[31] Nonselective beta-blockers are recommended to prevent bleeding in patients once varices are detected.[31]

Variceal hemorrhage, regardless of cirrhosis etiology, occurs at a rate of 5% to 15% per year.[32] Cirrhosis due to ALD (especially in the presence of continued drinking) is a major risk factor for progression from small to large varices and large varices are at higher risk of hemorrhage. Apart from size, other risk factors of hemorrhage are decompensated cirrhosis and endoscopic presence of red wale marks. Bleeding from esophageal varices is associated with a mortality rate of 20% at 6 weeks. Thus, it is vital that all patients with ALD should be aggressively screened to look for varices.[33] It is important to note that active alcohol consumption is a risk factor for precipitating esophageal variceal bleeding.

Gastric varices are less common when compared with esophageal varices and are seen in 5% to 33% of patients with portal hypertension.[34] Bleeding from gastric varices is reported in approximately 25% in 2 years. Risk factors for gastric variceal hemorrhage are similar to those of esophageal varices and include size, Child class and variceal red spots on endoscopy.[35]

Hepatocellular carcinoma

HCC generally occurs in patients with cirrhosis. There has been debate about whether patients with alcoholic cirrhosis have a lower risk of HCC and therefore might not need aggressive surveillance. Patients with alcoholic cirrhosis are likely have an HCC risk, which is equivalent to patients with other forms of cirrhosis (please see Joshi K, Kohli A, Manch R, et al: Alcoholic Liver Disease: High or Low risk for Developing Hepatocellular Carcinoma?, in this issue). Because of this increased risk of HCC in this population, surveillance is recommended. We believe that, in a general population with cirrhosis, the most effective surveillance strategy is to screen with alpha-fetoprotein (AFP) and ultrasound imaging every 6 months using the previously mentioned methods.[36,37] Some patients will require different forms of imaging to clarify findings on ultrasound. It should be noted that AFP is not recommended for HCC screening by the AASLD (American Association for the Study of Liver Diseases) guidelines.[38] The major issue with AFP is that it can be affected by the inflammatory status of the liver and therefore may not be reliable as an indicator of HCC. In our practice, we do use AFP cautiously to help screen for HCC, but only in combination with ultrasound.[39,40]

In contrast to patients with cirrhosis, as mentioned earlier, there is little consensus on whether noncirrhotic patients need to be screened for HCC or not.

It is hard to overemphasize the importance of regular office visits for patients who are at risk for the development of HCC. Patients and their families need to understand the lethal nature of HCC that can be successfully treated only with regular follow-up visits, routine HCC screening, and early detection.

Alcohol and Cancer, in General

In addition to the increased risk of liver cancer in patients with excessive alcohol intake and alcoholic cirrhosis, it must be remembered that excess alcohol consumption can increase the risk of multiple other cancers. Studies have shown that even small amounts of alcohol increase the risk for cancers of the oropharynx, esophagus, larynx, rectum, liver, and breast.[41–43] In the Million Women Study, the overall risk of cancer was increased 6% per consumption of 10 g alcohol per day of any type.[41] A large European study concluded that alcohol consumption could account for 10% of the attributable risk for any cancer in men, and 3% in women.[44] Even though no specific guidelines exist regarding the screening of patients with alcoholic cirrhosis for cancer (other than the HCC guidelines noted previously), it would seem prudent for the clinician to keep the increased risk of a multitude of cancers in mind when managing these patients. Also, the care provider should strongly recommend that the patient avoid smoking, given the increased risk of gastrointestinal and respiratory cancers in patients with combined alcohol and smoking.

Alcohol and Other Effects in the Body

Finally, although beyond the scope of this article, it must be recognized that alcohol abuse can contribute to many disease processes outside of the liver. Such processes can include chronic pancreatitis, and cardiomyopathy. The clinician must be aware of such issues in the long-term management of patients with chronic alcohol abuse and alcoholic cirrhosis.

SUMMARY

In conclusion, the most important role of the health care provider in the long-term management of the patient with ALD is to help ensure lifelong sobriety. This will require a commitment by the patient as well as potentially a multidisciplinary approach. Patients will need to be seen regularly in follow-up and screened for alcohol use. The role of pharmacotherapy to assist in the maintenance of abstinence is still not established.

Patients with ALD and cirrhosis are at risk for hepatic decompensation, portal hypertension, development of HCC, and a host of medical conditions brought on by the long-term toxic effects of alcohol. As outlined in this article, these need to be assessed and followed in these patients. Also, the effects of long-term alcohol abuse on other organ systems must be considered in the care of these patients.

REFERENCES

1. O'Shea RS, Dasarathy S, McCullough AJ, Practice Guideline Committee of the American Association for the Study of Liver Diseases, Practice Parameters Committee of the American College of Gastroenterology. Alcoholic liver disease. Hepatology 2010;51:307–28.
2. Kitchens JM. Does this patient have an alcohol problem? JAMA 1994;272(22): 1782–7.
3. World Health Organization. Evidence-based strategies and interventions to reduce alcohol-related harm. Global assessment of public-health problems caused by harmful use of alcohol; 60th World Health Assembly - A60/14 Add1. Geneva (Switzerland): World Health Organization; 2007.

4. U.S. Preventive Services Task Force. Screening and behavioral counseling interventions in primary care to reduce alcohol misuse: recommendation statement. Ann Intern Med 2004;140(7):554–6.

5. Girela E, Villanueva E, Hernandez-Cueto C, et al. Comparison of the CAGE questionnaire versus some biochemical markers in the diagnosis of alcoholism. Alcohol Alcohol 1994;29(3):337–43.

6. Aalto M, Seppä K. Use of laboratory markers and the audit questionnaire by primary care physicians to detect alcohol abuse by patients. Alcohol Alcohol 2005; 40(6):520–3.

7. Skinner HA, Sheu WJ. Reliability of alcohol use indices. The lifetime drinking history and the MAST. J Stud Alcohol 1982;43(11):1157–70.

8. Kenna GA, McGeary JE, Swift RM. Pharmacotherapy, pharmacogenomics, and the future of alcohol dependence treatment, part 1. Am J Health Syst Pharm 2004;61:2272–9.

9. Garbutt JC, Kranzler HR, O'Malley SS, et al. Efficacy and tolerability of long-acting injectable naltrexone for alcohol dependence: a randomized controlled trial. JAMA 2005;293:1617–25.

10. Rösner S, Hackl-Herrwerth A, Leucht S, et al. Acamprosate for alcohol dependence. Cochrane Database Syst Rev 2010;(9):CD004332.

11. Leone MA, Vigna-Taglianti F, Avanzi G, et al. Gammahydroxybutyrate (GHB) for treatment of alcohol withdrawal and prevention of relapses. Cochrane Database Syst Rev 2010;(2):CD006266.

12. Crabb DW. Pathogenesis of alcoholic liver disease: newer mechanisms of injury. Keio J Med 1999;48:184–8.

13. Leevy CM. Fatty liver: a study of 270 patients with biopsy proven fatty liver and review of the literature. Medicine (Baltimore) 1962;41:249–76.

14. Jaurigue MM, Cappell MS. Therapy for alcoholic liver disease. World J Gastroenterol 2014;20(9):2143–58.

15. Uchida T, Kao H, Quispe-Sjogren M, et al. Alcoholic foamy degeneration–a pattern of acute alcoholic injury of the liver. Gastroenterology 1983;84(4):683–92.

16. Bird GL. Investigation of alcoholic liver disease. Baillieres Clin Gastroenterol 1993;7:663–82.

17. Mathurin P, Poynard T, Ramond MJ, et al. Interet de la biopsie hepatique pour la selection des sujets suspects d'hepatitealcoolique aigue [Abstract]. Gastroenterol Clin Biol 1992;16:A231.

18. Bruha R, Dvorak K, Petrtyl J. Alcoholic liver disease. World J Hepatol 2012;4(3): 81–90.

19. Mendenhall CL, Anderson S, Weesner RE, et al. Protein-calorie malnutrition associated with alcoholic hepatitis. Veterans Administration Cooperative Study Group on Alcoholic Hepatitis. Am J Med 1984;76:211–22.

20. Mezey E. Interaction between alcohol and nutrition in the pathogenesis of alcoholic liver disease. Semin Liver Dis 1991;11:340–8.

21. Zenith L, Meena N, Ramadi A, et al. Eight weeks of exercise training increases aerobic capacity and muscle mass and reduces fatigue in patients with cirrhosis. Clin Gastroenterol Hepatol 2014;12(11):1920–6.e2.

22. de Franchis R. Updating consensus in portal hypertension: report of the Baveno III consensus workshop on definitions, methodology and therapeutic strategies in portal hypertension. J Hepatol 2000;33:846–52.

23. de Franchis R. Evolving Consensus in Portal Hypertension report of the Baveno IV consensus workshop on methodology of diagnosis and therapy in portal hypertension. J Hepatol 2005;43:167–76.

24. Wiest R, Groszmann RJ. Nitric oxide and portal hypertension: its role in the regulation of intrahepatic and splanchnic vascular resistance. Semin Liver Dis 2000; 19:411–26.
25. Sikuler E, Kravetz D, Groszmann RJ. Evolution of portal hypertension and mechanisms involved in its maintenance in a rat model. Am J Physiol 1985;248(6 Pt 1): G618–25.
26. Pagliaro L, D'Amico G, Pasta L, et al. Portal hypertension in cirrhosis: natural history. In: Bosch J, Groszmann RJ, editors. Portal hypertension. Pathophysiology and treatment. Oxford (United Kingdom): Blackwell Scientific; 1994. p. 72–92.
27. Merli M, Nicolini G, Angeloni S, et al. Incidence and natural history of small esophageal varices in cirrhotic patients. J Hepatol 2003;38:266–72.
28. Groszmann RJ, Garcia-Tsao G, Bosch J, et al, Portal Hypertension Collaborative Group. Beta-blockers to prevent gastroesophageal varices in patients with cirrhosis. N Engl J Med 2005;353:2254–61.
29. Casado M, Bosch J, Garcia-Pagan JC, et al. Clinical events after transjugular intrahepatic portosystemic shunt: correlation with hemodynamic findings. Gastroenterology 1998;114:1296–303.
30. Grace ND, Groszmann RJ, Garcia-Tsao G, et al. Portal hypertension and variceal bleeding: an AASLD single topic symposium. Hepatology 1998;28:868–80.
31. D'Amico G, Garcia-Tsao G, Cales P, et al. Diagnosis of portal hypertension: how and when. In: de Franchis R, editor. Portal Hypertension III. Proceedings of the Third Baveno International Consensus Workshop on Definitions, Methodology and Therapeutic Strategies. Oxford (United Kingdom): Blackwell Science; 2001. p. 36–64.
32. The North Italian Endoscopic Club for the Study and Treatment of Esophageal Varices. Prediction of the first variceal hemorrhage in patients with cirrhosis of the liver and esophageal varices. A prospective multicenter study. N Engl J Med 1988;319:983–9.
33. D'Amico G, de Franchis R. Upper digestive bleeding in cirrhosis. Posttherapeutic outcome and prognostic indicators. Hepatology 2003;38:599–612.
34. Sarin SK, Lahoti D, Saxena SP, et al. Prevalence, classification and natural history of gastric varices: a long-term follow-up study in 568 portal hypertension patients. Hepatology 1992;16:1343–9.
35. Kim T, Shijo H, Kokawa H, et al. Risk factors for hemorrhage from gastric fundal varices. Hepatology 1997;25:307–12.
36. Thompson Coon J, Rogers G, Hewson P, et al. Surveillance of cirrhosis for hepatocellular carcinoma: systematic review and economic analysis. Health Technol Assess 2007;11(34):1–206.
37. Kanwal F, Kramer J, Asch SM, et al. An explicit quality indicator set for measurement of quality of care in patients with cirrhosis. Clin Gastroenterol Hepatol 2010; 8(8):709–17.
38. Bruix J, Sherman M, American Association for the Study of Liver Diseases. Management of hepatocellular carcinoma: an update. Hepatology 2010;53:1020–2.
39. El-Serag HB, Mason AC. Rising incidence of hepatocellular carcinoma in the United States. N Engl J Med 1999;340(10):745–50.
40. Deuffic S, Poynard T, Buffat L, et al. Trends in primary liver cancer. Lancet 1998; 351(9097):214–5.
41. Allen NE, Beral V, Casabonne D, et al. Moderate alcohol intake and cancer incidence in women. J Natl Cancer Inst 2009;101(5):296.
42. Zhang SM, Lee IM, Manson JE, et al. Alcohol consumption and breast cancer risk in the Women's Health Study. Am J Epidemiol 2007;165(6):667.

43. Chen WY, Rosner B, Hankinson SE, et al. Moderate alcohol consumption during adult life, drinking patterns, and breast cancer risk. JAMA 2011;306(17):1884.
44. Schutze M, Boeing H, Pischon T, et al. Alcohol attributable burden of incidence of cancer in eight European countries based on results from prospective cohort study. BMJ 2011;342:1584.

Alcoholic Liver Disease

High Risk or Low Risk for Developing Hepatocellular Carcinoma?

Kartik Joshi, MBS, BS[a], Anita Kohli, MD, MS[a,b], Richard Manch, MD[a],
Robert Gish, MD[a,c],*

KEYWORDS

- Alcoholic liver disease • Hepatocellular carcinoma risk • Cirrhosis • Hepatitis B
- Hepatitis C • Diabetes • Obesity

KEY POINTS

- Although the evidence has been conflicting, it seems that the linkage between alcoholic liver disease (ALD)–associated compensated cirrhosis and hepatocellular carcinoma (HCC) is best characterized as medium–high risk.
- Alcohol interacts with other causes of liver disease, including hepatitis B and C, and conditions, such as diabetes and obesity, to increase the risk for developing HCC, either synergistically or additively.
- HCC risk in patients with ALD-associated cirrhosis increases with age and with quantity and duration of alcohol consumption and is pronounced in women.

INTRODUCTION

In the United States, alcoholic liver disease (ALD) is the second leading cause of liver transplantation and cirrhosis behind chronic infection with hepatitis C virus (HCV).[1–3] Globally, alcohol accounts for 50% of all deaths due to cirrhosis.[4] The clinical spectrum of ALD includes steatosis, sclerosing hyaline necrosis, acute on chronic liver failure, alcoholic hepatitis, cirrhosis, and hepatocellular carcinoma (HCC). Although the prevalence of ALD-associated cirrhosis (defined here as cirrhosis that develops exclusively as the result of alcohol intake, with no other contributing factors) is high globally,

The authors have nothing to disclose.
[a] Division of Hepatology, St. Joseph's Hospital and Medical Center, Creighton University School of Medicine, 500 West Thomas Road, Suite 900, Phoenix, AZ 85013, USA; [b] Division of Infectious Disease, St. Joseph's Hospital and Medical Center, Creighton University School of Medicine, 500 West Thomas Road, Suite 900, Phoenix, AZ 85013, USA; [c] Division of Hepatology and Gastroenterology, Stanford University Hospitals and Clinics, 300 Pasteur Drive, Palo Alto, CA 94304, USA
* Corresponding author. 6022 La Jolla Mesa Drive, La Jolla, CA 92037.
E-mail address: rgish@robertgish.com

Clin Liver Dis 20 (2016) 563–580
http://dx.doi.org/10.1016/j.cld.2016.02.012   liver.theclinics.com
1089-3261/16/$ – see front matter © 2016 The Authors. Published by Elsevier Inc. This is an open access article under the CC BY-NC-ND license (http://creativecommons.org/licenses/by-nc-nd/4.0/).

the incidence of HCC associated with alcoholic cirrhosis is lower than the incidence associated with cirrhosis of other etiologies, including chronic HCV, chronic hepatitis B virus (HBV), and hereditary hemochromatosis.[5] To better understand the relationship between ALD and the development of HCC, several studies have investigated alcohol as the primary cause and as a cofactor for carcinogenesis along with other etiologies of liver disease, such as viral hepatitis, hemochromatosis, and fatty liver disease. Additionally, studies have shown that host factors such as gender, genetics, and ethnicity may influence disease progression. This review critically assesses the literature to evaluate the risk posed by alcohol as a primary cause of and as a cofactor for the development of HCC.

AS A PRIMARY CAUSE: THE RISK OF HEPATOCELLULAR CARCINOMA IN PATIENTS WITH ALCOHOLIC LIVER DISEASE–ASSOCIATED CIRRHOSIS

There have been conflicting findings on the level of HCC risk in patients with compensated ALD-associated cirrhosis. Seven studies evaluating HCC risk in patients with cirrhosis associated exclusively with alcohol consumption (with no evidence of ongoing viral hepatitis infection) have suggested that the 10-year cumulative incidence may range from 6.8-28.7%.[6–12] In some of these studies, patients with ALD-associated cirrhosis were evaluated alongside patients with chronic hepatitis B (CHB)- and chronic hepatitis C (CHC)-associated cirrhosis.[6,9,11,12] (**Tables 1** and **2**).

Table 1 Summary of key studies investigating hepatocellular carcinoma risk for patients with compensated alcoholic cirrhosis (without concomitant viral hepatitis)						
Study	Country	Total Patients (n)	Follow-up (y)	Age (y)	Male/ Female	Hepatocellular Carcinoma Cumulative Incidence
Toshikuni et al,[6] 2009	Japan	227	3.5[b]	59[b]	67/8	Annual: 0.6% 3-y: 1.3% 5-y: 6.8% 7-y: 6.8% 10-y: 6.8%
Jepsen et al,[7] 2012	Demark	8482	4.1[b]	54.4[b]	5655/2827	5-y: 1.0%
Ioannou et al,[11] 2007	USA	2126	3.6[a]	NA	2062/64	0.6/100 Patient-years
Uetake et al,[8] 2003	Japan	91	5.9[b]	50.1[b]	91/0	3-y: 2.4% 5-y: 6.4% 7-y: 18.9% 10-y: 28.7%
N'Kontchou et al,[9] 2006	France	771	4.1[a]	59.7[a]	336/142	5-y: 16%
Mancebo et al,[10] 2013	Spain	450	3.5[b]	53.9[a]	369/81	Annual: 2.6% 5-y: 13.2% 10-y: 23.2%
Lin et al,[12] 2013	Taiwan	966	5.2[a]	49.3[b]	165/37	Annual: 1.9% 3-y: 4.8% 5-y: 8.9% 10-y: 21.4%

[a] Mean.
[b] Median.

Evidence Suggesting Patients with Alcoholic Cirrhosis are at Low Risk for Hepatocellular Carcinoma

Two of the studies outlined in **Table 1** evaluated the risk of HCC in patients with ALD-associated cirrhosis and suggested that the risk is low. With subgroup analysis, however, certain categories of patients are shown to have higher HCC risk. A large retrospective population-based study of 8482 Danish patients with ALD-associated cirrhosis found a 5-year cumulative risk for developing HCC of 1%.[7] A stratified analysis, however, found several demographic groups who exhibited a higher risk for developing HCC. Men (n = 5,655) had a 5-year risk of 1.5% (95% CI, 12–1.8) which was several-fold greater than the 5-year risk for women (n = 2,827) of 0.2% (95% CI, 0.1–0.4). Additionally, the risk for developing HCC increased with age. Approximately 33% of the cohort was less than 50 years old and had a 5-year HCC risk of 0.3% (95% CI, 0.1–0.5). In contrast, patients who were greater than or equal to 70 years old had a nearly 6.5-fold greater risk of 1.9% (95% CI, 1.0–3.3). In addition, an analysis of a subset of patients (n = 320) whose diagnosis of cirrhosis was corroborated by additional chart reviews and who were followed up by hepatologists found the 5-year HCC risk to be 1.9%. This was nearly double that of the primary group, suggesting a potential misclassification bias of the primary cohort and an underestimation of HCC risk.

Another retrospective study of 2,126 cirrhotic patients seen at United States Veterans Affairs centers evaluated the incidence and predictors of HCC.[11] Among the 734 patients (35% of the population) with ALD-associated cirrhosis, the aggregate HCC incidence was only 0.6 per 100 patient-years. In contrast, patients with chronic HBV-associated and chronic HCV-associated cirrhosis had HCC incidence rates of 2.4 and 3.6 per 100 patient years, respectively. Because of its scale and design, this study was able to identify seven risk factors for the development of HCC in cirrhotics and adjust for key confounding variables. Ultimately, HCC incidence rates changed more than 20-fold depending on the presence of other risk factors evaluated in the study: CHC, hepatitis B surface antigen (HBsAg), hepatitis B core antibody (anti-HBc), obesity, overweight, diabetes, and gradations of low platelets (**Table 2**). Significantly, alcohol only, as a cause of cirrhosis, was not implicated as a risk factor for HCC.

Evidence Suggesting Patients with Alcoholic Cirrhosis are at Medium–High Risk for Hepatocellular Carcinoma

Conversely, the other 5 studies outlined in **Table 1** suggest that patients with ALD-associated cirrhosis are at a medium–high risk (10-year cumulative risk 21.4%–28.7%) for the development of HCC.[6,8–10,12] A prospective cohort study following 91 Japanese males with compensated alcoholic cirrhosis who were HBsAg-negative and anti-HCV-negative reported a 6.4% (5-year) and 28.7% (10-year) cumulative incidence of HCC.[8] In comparing alcoholic cirrhotic patients with (n = 13) and without (n = 78) HCC, two critical differences were observed. Those with HCC had a far greater lifetime cumulative alcohol consumption (P = .0047) and were more likely to have been exposed to HBV (P = .0598) as evidenced by the presence of anti-HBc. The 3, 5, 7, and 10-year cumulative incidence rates of HCC were 8.4%, 19.9%, 33.2%, and 41.6% in the subset of alcoholic cirrhotics whose cumulative alcohol consumption exceeded 1200 kg compared to 0%, 2.0%, 10.8%, and 20.7%, respectively, in patients with a cumulative alcohol consumption less than 1200 kg.

Similarly, a prospective cohort study following 478 patients with well-compensated ALD-associated cirrhosis without viral hepatitis found a medium risk for developing HCC.[9] N'Kontchou and colleagues reported a 5-year HCC cumulative incidence rate of 16% and identified four independent predictors of HCC in alcoholic cirrhotics: age

Table 2
Comparison of the effects of risk factors on the development of hepatocellular carcinoma in patients with cirrhosis

Study	Study Design	Risk Factors Evaluated	Reference Point	Hazard Ratio (HR)/Odds Ratio (OR)/Relative Risk (RR)/Regression Coefficient (RC)	95% CI	P value
Chung et al,[38] 2007	Retrospective	*HCC risk*				
		HBV and ethanol cirrhosis	Ethanol-only cirrhosis	OR 17.609		P = .001
		HBV cirrhosis		OR 8.449	NR	P = .001
		Age		OR 1.056		P = .001
Donato et al,[20] 2002	Case-control[a]	*HCC risk*				
		HBV (–), HCV (–), consumes >60 g/d	HBV (–) and HCV (–) and consumes 0–60 g/d	OR 7.0	4.5–11.1	
		HBV (+), consumes 0–60 g/d		OR 22.8	12.1–42.8	
		HBV (+), consumes >60 g/d		OR 48.6	24.1–98.0	NR
		HCV (+), consumes 0–60 g/d		OR 55.0	29.9–101	
		HCV (+), consumes >60 g/d		OR 109	50.9–233	
Wang et al,[39] 2003	Population-based cohort	*HCC risk*		RR		
		Age	Age: 30–39			
		40–49		4.39	1.90–10.14	
		50–59		9.22	4.20–20.24	
		60+		9.63	4.16–22.28	
		Residence: Penghu Islets	Residence: Taiwan Island	RR 2.06	1.41–3.00	
		HBsAg serostatus: (+)	(–) HBsAg	RR 13.14	8.60–20.08	
		Anti-HCV serostatus: (+)	(–) Anti-HCV	RR 2.45	1.42–4.22	
		Years of schooling	× <6 y of schooling	RR		
		6		0.75	0.45–1.25	
		× >6		0.72	0.41–1.28	NR
		Ethnicity	Ethnicity: Fukienese	RR		
		Hakka		1.66	0.94–2.94	
		China Mainlander/aborigine		0.80	0.39–1.67	
		Cigarette smoking: yes	No cigarette smoking	RR 1.55	1.06–2.26	
		Duration of cigarette smoking (y)	Nonsmokers	RR		
		1–25		0.98	0.54–1.77	
		× >25		1.91	1.25–2.91	

Alcohol drinking: yes	No alcohol drinking	RR 1.46	0.97–2.21	
Duration of alcohol drinking (y)	Nondrinkers	RR		
1–20		1.34	0.64–2.79	
× >20		1.56	0.95–2.55	
Betel quid chewing: yes	No betel quid chewing	RR 1.59	0.89–2.85	
Quantity betel quid chewed/d	Nonchewer	RR		
1–10		1.44	0.66–3.14	
× >10		1.92	0.87–4.22	
No. substance use habits	0 Substance abuse habits	RR		
1		1.36	0.88–2.01	
2		1.60	0.95–2.70	
3		3.15	1.45–6.89	
Familial history HCC (1st-degree relatives): yes	No familial HCC history (1st-degree relatives)	RR 1.46	0.68–3.15	
Liver function at recruitment (AST >30 or ALT >35): dysfunction	Normal liver function at recruitment	RR 3.15	2.13–4.67	
Tagger et al,[46] 1999	Case-control[b]	HCC risk		
HCV RNA (+) and ethanol	HCV RNA (−) and ethanol	OR		
0–40 g/d	0–40 g/d	26.1	12.6–54.0	
41–80 g/d		62.6	23.3–168	
× >80 g/d		126	42.8–373	
HCV RNA (+) and HBsAg (−)	HCV RNA (−) and HBsAg (−)	OR 35.6	14.5–87.1	
HCV RNA (−) and HBsAg (+)	—	OR 21.1	11.1–40.0	
HCV RNA (+) and HBsAg (+)	—	OR 132	15.3–890	
HCV RNA (−) and anti-HBs (+), anti-HBc (+) or anti-HBs (+) alone	—	OR 1.3	0.8–2.1	NR
HCV RNA (+) and anti-HBs (+), anti-HBc (+) or anti-HBs (+) alone	—	OR 36.5	16.0–83.1	
HCV RNA (−) and anti-HBc (+)	—	OR 1.7	1.0–2.9	
HCV RNA (+) and anti-HBc (+)	—	OR 29.8	10.9–56.8	

(continued on next page)

Table 2
(continued)

Study	Study Design	Risk Factors Evaluated	Reference Point	Hazard Ratio (HR)/ Odds Ratio (OR)/ Relative Risk (RR)/Regression Coefficient (RC)	95% CI	P value
Tsutsumi et al,[47] 1996	Retrospective	*HCC risk for the following causes of cirrhosis*				
		Ethanol	No evidence of HBV, HCV, or alcohol in developing cirrhosis or HCC	OR 1.22	NR	NR
		HBV		OR 4.49		
		HCV		OR 2.39		
		HBV + ethanol		OR 4.96		
		HCV + ethanol		OR 5.28		
		HBV + HCV		OR 3.01		
Miyakawa et al,[67] 1993	Retrospective	*HCC risk*				
		Ethanol cirrhosis	NR	OR 0.615	NR	NS
		HCV cirrhosis		OR 1.90		P<.05
		HCV and ethanol Cirrhosis		OR 3.65		P<.01
		Child-Pugh A		OR 0.653		P<.05
		Male gender		OR 2.06		P<.01
Uetake et al,[8] 2003	Prospective	*HCC risk in ethanol cirrhotics (without HBV or HCV)*				
		Cumulative alcohol intake	NR	RC 0.0017; Z 2.83	NR	P = .0047
		(+) Anti-HBc		RC 1.1533; Z 1.88		P = .0598
Aizawa et al,[44] 2000	Retrospective	*HCC risk in chronic HCV patients*				
		Age ≥50	Age <50	RR 4.54	2.06-9.98	P = .0002
		Male gender	Female gender	RR 2.80	0.92-8.52	P = .07
		Ethanol consumption 65 g/d >5 y (habitual heavy drinking)	No habitual heavy drinking	RR 3.04	1.31-7.09	P = .01
		Minimum ALT ≥40	ALT, 40	RR 1.80	0.84-3.87	P = .13
		IFN therapy	No IFN therapy	RR 0.78	0.30-1.98	P = .596
		Staging (severe fibrosis)	Mild staging	RR 3.48	1.51-8.06	P = .004
		Irregular regeneration (severe)	Mild regeneration	RR 1.19	0.45-3.20	P = .724

Study	Design	Risk factor		Estimate	95% CI	P value
Ioannou et al,[11] 2007	Retrospective	*HCC risk in cirrhotics*				
		HCV	NR	HR 3.0	1.7–5.3	
		HBsAg		HR 3.3	1.4–7.7	
		Anti-HBc		HR 1.7	1.1–2.8	
		BMI	BMI <25	HR		
		25–30		2.8	1.5–5.4	
		≥30		2.5	1.3–4.9	NR
		Diabetes	NR	HR 1.5	0.9–2.5	
		Platelet count	Platelet count >266	HR		
		180–266		2.1	0.8–5.6	
		111–179		3.3	1.3–8.0	
		× <111		4.7	2.0–11.4	
Kwon et al,[41] 2012	Case-control[c]	*HCC risk*				
		(+) Anti-HBc	Patients with cirrhosis	OR 3.1	1.354–7.098	P = .007
		(+) Anti-HBc and (+) anti-HBs	and anti-HBc (−)	OR 2.61	1.090–6.287	P = .031
		(+) Anti-HBc and (−) anti-HBs		OR 4.16	1.571–11.01	P = .004
		(+) Anti-HBc and (−) HBV DNA		OR 2.7	1.12–6.49	P = .027
		(+) Anti-HBc and (+) HBV DNA		OR 3.13	1.11–8.81	P = .039
Mancebo et al,[10] 2013	Prospective	*HCC risk in ethanol cirrhotics*				
		Age ≥55	NR	HR 2.39	1.27–4.51	P = .007
		Platelets <125		HR 3.29	1.39–7.85	P = .007
N'Kontchou et al,[9] 2006	Prospective	*HCC risk in cirrhotics (HCV, ethanol, HCV + ethanol)*				
		Age	Age: <50	HR		
		50–60		1.6	0.9–2.9	P = NS
		60–70		2.4	1.3–4.3	P = .005
		>70		3.0	1.7–5.5	P<.0001
		Male gender	Gender: female	HR 2.0	1.4–2.7	P<.0001
		Cirrhosis cause	Cirrhosis cause: ethanol	HR		
		HCV		1.6	1.2–2.2	P = .002
		HCV and ethanol		2.6	1.7–4.0	P<.0001
		BMI	BMI: <25	HR		
		25–30		2.0	14–2.7	P<.0001
		≥30		2.8	2.0–4.0	P<.0001
		Diabetes	Diabetes: no	HR 1.6	1.2–2.1	P = .001

(continued on next page)

Table 2
(continued)

Study	Study Design	Risk Factors Evaluated	Reference Point	Hazard Ratio (HR)/ Odds Ratio (OR)/ Relative Risk (RR)/Regression Coefficient (RC)	95% CI	P value
Marrero et al,[66] 2005	Case-control[c]	*HCC risk*	*Cirrhotic patients*			
		Alcohol (gram-years)	Alcohol: none	OR		
		<1500		0.5	0.1–0.7	
		≥1500		5.7	2.4–13.7	
		Tobacco (pack-years)	Tobacco: none	OR		NR
		<20		0.7	0.4–1.2	
		≥20		4.9	2.2–10.6	
		BMI	Obesity: lean	OR		
		25.1–30		0.3	0.09–0.5	
		≥30		4.3	2.1–8.4	
Loomba et al,[65] 2010	Prospective	*HCC risk in REVEAL-HBV cohort*				
		BMI and ethanol usage	BMI <30 and no ethanol use	BMI and ethanol usage	BMI and ethanol usage	BMI and ethanol usage
		BMI ≥30, no use		HR 0.64	0.16–2.63	P = .5385
		BMI <30, yes use		HR 1.64	1.12–2.40	P = .0106
		BMI ≥30, yes use		HR 3.40	1.24–9.34	P = .0176

Abbreviations: NR, not reported; NS, not significant.
[a] Controls did not have liver disease, although consumed alcohol.
[b] Controls did not have HCV or HBV; Number with cirrhosis not reported.
[c] Controls were cirrhosis (+) and HCC (−).

>70, male gender, having a BMI ≥30, and diabetes (see **Table 2**). Similar to other studies, this study did not report any data on volume of alcohol consumption. Likewise, a prospective study following 450 patients with compensated ALD-associated cirrhosis reported an annual HCC incidence of 2.6%, along with 5 and 10-year cumulative rates of 13.2% and 23.2%, respectively.[10] Multivariate analysis identified two independent risk factors for developing HCC, age ≥55 and having a platelet count less than 125 (see **Table 2**). Based on the presence or absence of these critical factors, the HCC risk varied dramatically. Patients who lacked both risk factors (n = 93) had an annual HCC incidence of 0.3% compared to 2.6% in those with one risk factor (n = 228) and 4.8% in those with both risk factors (n = 129). To ensure the validity of these findings, the same analysis was performed in a subset of 140 patients with histologically confirmed alcoholic cirrhosis. Similar annual incidences of HCC were observed: 0%, 2.7%, and 3.4% for patients with 0, 1, and 2 risk factors, respectively.

A retrospective cohort study of Japanese patients with compensated cirrhosis observed annual and 5-year cumulative incidence rates of 0.6% and 6.8%, respectively. Additionally, this study reported 10-year HCC cumulative incidence rates that were approximately 7.5 fold higher in patients with CHC-associated cirrhosis (n = 152) compared to those with ALD-associated cirrhosis, 50.3% and 6.8%, respectively (*P* = .0003).[6] Finally, a Taiwanese retrospective cohort study following 966 cirrhotic patients further reinforced the notion that ALD-associated cirrhosis poses a more than modest risk for the development of HCC.[12] The study cohort consisted of patients with three etiologies of cirrhosis: CHB alone (n = 632), combined CHB and alcohol (n = 132) and alcohol alone (n = 202). Within the alcoholic cirrhosis subset, among the 110 patients who were Child-Pugh Grade A the annual, 5-year, and 10-year HCC incidence rates were 1.9%, 8.9%, and 21.4%. The aforementioned incidence rates were all higher when patients with decompensated alcoholic-cirrhosis, Child-Pugh Grades A-C, were included.

In summary, the interpretation of findings from these key studies is complicated by the heterogeneity in study design, especially with respect to patient populations analyzed (beyond cause), mixed causes of liver cirrhosis, evaluation of liver fibrosis, definition of liver cirrhosis, utilization of HCC surveillance, adjustments for key confounding variables, and the extent to which alcohol consumption was assessed (see **Table 1**). Nevertheless, there is solid support for a medium-high risk linkage between ALD and HCC, with risk increasing with age, cumulative lifetime alcohol consumption, and the presence of additional causes of liver disease. A more refined risk determination for the development of HCC can be readily achieved by incorporating the risk factors reported in many studies (see **Table 2**). The use of these findings to manage HCC risk for patients with ALD-associated cirrhosis is particularly important because of the paucity of evidence on the use of biomarkers, such as α-fetoprotein (AFP) , α-fetoprotein–L3 (AFP-L3), and des-gamma carboxyprothrombin (DCP) for HCC surveillance in this patient population.[13] Ultimately, to develop a comprehensive understanding of alcohol and its relationship to HCC, it is necessary to also examine the interaction of alcohol and HCC with different host factors, etiologies of liver disease, and comorbidities.

ALCOHOL CONSUMPTION PATTERNS AND HOST FACTORS

Although quantity and duration of alcohol consumption have been associated with ALD progression[14] and an increased risk for developing HCC,[15] not all patients who chronically overconsume alcohol develop alcoholic cirrhosis and/or HCC. Instead, progression to ALD is influenced by the interaction between consumption and a constellation of host factors, leading to the development of cirrhosis and HCC in only a subset of patients.

Alcohol Consumption and Alcoholic Liver Disease Risk: Dose Dependent or Threshold Effect?

Many studies have investigated whether a discrete threshold of consumption or dose dependence characterizes the relationship between alcohol consumption and the development of cirrhosis and/or HCC. Some studies have suggested that a threshold delineating safe alcohol consumption from risky behavior may exist.[16,17] A retrospective study of 210 deceased males found that consumption less than 40 g per day over a 25-year period did not increase the incidence of ALD. Other studies have suggested that this threshold may be lower. A population-based, cross-sectional study surveying 2 northern Italian towns found that the risk threshold for developing cirrhosis was greater than 30 g per day, equivalent to a lifetime intake of 100 kg.[17] In this study, the lower risk threshold was independent of gender and the risk of cirrhosis below this threshold was minimal. A meta-analysis found an even lower threshold for cirrhosis development of 25 g per day.[18]

Conversely, other studies have found evidence of a dose-response relationship between alcohol consumption and the development of cirrhosis.[19–21] In a large-scale prospective population study, a dose-dependent curve emerged for the development of alcohol-induced cirrhosis in men and women.[19] Women had a higher risk for developing cirrhosis at a lower intake than men, with increased risk seen at a weekly consumption of 84 g to 156 g compared with 168 g to 324 g for men. A similar trend was seen for the development of HCC in a hospital-based case-control study (n = 464 HCC patients) where women had a nearly 5-fold higher risk for developing HCC with heavy alcohol consumption of greater than 80 g per day (adjusted OR 7.5).[20]

There does not seem to be a level of alcohol intake that absolutely equates with cirrhosis in all people. In the Dionysos Study, a large cohort study of the prevalence of chronic liver disease in the general population of two northern Italian communities that included 6,534 people free of virus-related chronic liver disease, at the lowest level of intake found to be associated with either cirrhosis or non-cirrhotic liver damage (NCLD), more than 30 g per day, 2.2% became cirrhotic and 3.3% showed persistent signs of NCLD; at the highest level of consumption, more than120 g per day, only 13.5% either developed cirrhosis or showed signs of liver damage.[17]

In summary, there is likely neither a strict, linear dose-dependent relationship nor is there a universally accepted threshold that characterizes the relationship between alcohol consumption and the risk for developing cirrhosis and/or HCC. Evidence suggests, however, that the risk increases appreciably, albeit at different rates for each gender, when consumption exceeds certain levels. The magnitude of this increased risk remains difficult to ascertain for two structural reasons. For one, some influential case-control studies utilized healthy controls[20] which often contributes to an overestimation of risk.[22] Additionally, multiple meta-analyses have reported, and to some extent quantified, the effects of heterogeneity in study design, study endpoint, and geographic area of study on risk estimates.[15,18,21]

Drinking Patterns: With or Without a Meal

Multiple studies have shown that the risk for developing alcoholic cirrhosis and ALD is increased when alcohol is consumed without any accompanying food.[17,23] Bellentani and colleagues[17] found an OR of 3.4 (95% CI, 1.7–6.6) favoring the development of cirrhosis when drinking outside of a meal. Similarly, a population-based study in China found that those who drank without food were 2.7 times more likely to develop ALD. It is likely that this increased risk can be explained by differences in absorption and volume of distribution. To date, no study has directly evaluated the risk of developing HCC from consuming alcohol with or without food.

The Effect of Abstinence on the Risk of Cirrhosis and Hepatocellular Carcinoma

Paradoxically, multiple studies have shown that patients with alcoholic cirrhosis who abstain from further alcohol consumption are at a higher risk for developing HCC than ongoing drinkers at the same intake levels.[20,24] This counterintuitive finding might be explained by considering the often large degree of liver damage that has developed by the time a patient completely and permanently abstains from alcohol; the profound damage to the liver parenchyma is often a precursor to irreversible disease progression and/or HCC.

Evidence also exists, however, suggesting that with sufficient time after cessation of alcohol consumption, the risk of developing HCC in abstaining patients with ALD-associated cirrhosis can eventually approach the risk faced by those who have never consumed alcohol. In a comprehensive meta-analysis, Heckley and colleagues[25] showed that the risk of developing HCC may drop by as much as 6% to 7% per year after abstinence is begun. Even more encouraging, after 23 years of continued abstinence, the risk of developing HCC may normalize and become equivalent to the level faced by someone who has never consumed alcohol. However, the authors from this important study warn that this estimate has a high degree of statistical uncertainty, as evidenced by the wide 95% confidence interval for the time scale needed to achieve a normalized risk for HCC.

Gender and Hormones

Women are at a higher risk for developing cirrhosis and HCC at lower levels of alcohol consumption than their male counterparts. Some evidence suggests this higher risk for developing cirrhosis remains for women even during abstinence.[26] In a seminal study, it was found that not only do female ALD patients develop fibrosis earlier, they also experience a more rapid progression toward cirrhosis compared to males (20 years vs 35 years; $P<.001$).[27] There are key biochemical differences between men and women such as first-pass metabolism, volume of distribution, and gastric alcohol dehydrogenase kinetics that are suspected to partially explain the higher risk faced by women.[28–30] Additionally, hormones and endocrine changes may play a role as possible cofactors in the pathogenesis of ALD.[31] Although limited evidence exists in clinical studies, animal models have shown that estrogen is linked with the sensitization of Kupffer cells to endotoxins and eventually to increased tumor necrosis factor α synthesis.[32–34] It is suspected that these processes likely contribute to the milieu that may lead to the development of severe ALD in women.

Race and Ethnicity

Limited evidence exists supporting a greater prevalence of ALD-associated cirrhosis in particular ethnic groups, namely South Asian males.[35] More studies are needed to understand to what extent any differences can be attributed to cultural factors,[36] genetics, consumption patterns, or access to medical care.

ALCOHOL AS A COFACTOR WITH OTHER CAUSES OF LIVER DISEASE FOR HEPATOCELLULAR CARCINOMA DEVELOPMENT

Hepatitis B: Chronic or Occult

Multiple studies have shown that alcohol is a cofactor that acts synergistically with chronic HBV to increase the risk and incidence of developing HCC.[12,20,37–39] In a Taiwanese retrospective cohort study comparing HCC risk among patients with different etiologies of cirrhosis (chronic HBV only, alcohol only, and combined chronic HBV and alcohol), cirrhotic patients with chronic HBV and alcoholism, defined as consuming more than 80 g per day of alcohol over a 5-year period, had the highest annual and 10-year cumulative incidences of developing HCC at 9.9% and 52.8%, respectively.[12] Additionally, patients with combined chronic HBV and alcoholism developed HCC at a younger age compared with cirrhotics of chronic HBV-only or alcoholism-only etiologies (43.9 years, 47.8 years, 49.3 years, respectively; P = .03). However, the combined chronic HBV and alcoholism group had a higher proportion of patients with decompensated liver disease, Child-Pugh grades B and C (54%), compared with the chronic HBV-only (43%) and alcoholism-only (46%) groups.

Studies have also suggested that occult HBV infection (defined as a state in which there is loss of HBsAg; intrahepatic persistence of entire, episomal, replication-competent HBV genomes, such as HBV covalently closed circular DNA chromatinized episomes; detectable HBV DNA in the liver; and phases of undetectable and very low but detectable HBV DNA in serum and in some cases HBV serum markers that are all negative[40]) might be a risk factor for developing HCC.[8,41] In a case-control study of 144 HBsAg-negative Korean men with ALD-associated cirrhosis, 72 diagnosed with HCC matched by age to 72 without, it was found that anti-HBc positivity was the only risk factor for developing HCC (odds ratio [OR] 3.1; 95% CI, 1.354–7.098; P = .007).[41] Similarly, a prospective cohort study of 91 Japanese patients with alcoholic cirrhosis found that patients who were anti-HBc positive but HBsAg negative had a greater cumulative incidence and overall likelihood of developing HCC compared with those who were anti-HBc negative (P = .015).[8] The HCC occurrence rates in 31 patients with and 60 patients without anti-HBc were 15.6% and 2.9% at 5 years, 28.4% and 13.5% at 7 years, and 40.4% and 22.1% at 10 years, respectively.

Chronic Hepatitis C

Multiple studies have shown that consumption of alcohol in the presence of chronic HCV is associated with disease progression[42–45] along with an increased risk for developing cirrhosis and HCC.[9,46,47] A prospective cohort study found that patients with combined chronic HCV–alcoholic cirrhosis had a higher risk of developing HCC (hazard ratio [HR] 2.6; 95% CI, 1.7–4.0) than patients with chronic HCV-only cirrhosis or alcoholic-only cirrhosis.[9] Akin to chronic HBV, studies have found that a synergistic relationship exists between alcohol and chronic HCV in increasing the risk for developing HCC.[46,47] An Italian case-control study found that the synergistic interaction increased with the intake level of alcohol.[46]

Hereditary Hemochromatosis

Although the fundamental genetics of hemochromatosis have been largely identified with key discoveries such as the HFE gene, its expression remains somewhat enigmatic, given its incomplete penetration. As such, the phenotype of hereditary hemochromatosis is dependent on the interaction between genetics and multiple environmental factors, most notably gender, age, and alcohol. In a retrospective study of 378 patients homozygous for the C282Y mutation, daily alcohol consumption greater than or equal to 60 g was associated with greater abnormalities in iron and liver biochemical values, including greater serum ferritin, alanine aminotransferase (ALT), and aspartate aminotransferase (AST) values (P<.001) along with higher iron and transferrin saturation (P<.01) compared to their counterparts whose daily alcohol consumption was less than 60 g.[48] Furthermore, an Australian study of 224 patients homozygous for the C282Y mutation found that patients whose alcohol consumption exceeded 60 g per day had an 8.7-fold greater prevalence of cirrhosis compared with their counterparts who drank less than 60 g per day (P<.001).[49] Significantly, the average level of hepatic iron concentration at which cirrhosis developed was lower (mean = 406 μmol/g compared to mean = 271 μmol/g) in the subset who consumed more alcohol (P = .045). In addition, cirrhosis occurred at an earlier age in the group with higher alcohol consumption, at an average age of 46.5 years compared with 53.7 years (P = .048). Interestingly, similar findings were also seen when the analysis was repeated using a lower quantity of alcohol, 40 g per day.

Genetics and Polymorphisms

With the advances in genomics and molecular biology techniques, several studies have found associations between genetic polymorphisms and ALD. Most prominent and agreed upon are the polymorphisms in the patatin-like phospholipase domain-containing protein 3 (PNPLA3) gene, a highly expressed protein in the liver involved in lipid metabolism, although its exact function remains unknown. Increasingly, there is evidence linking single-nucleotide polymorphisms (SNPs) in the PNPLA3 gene to a possible predisposition to ALD, along with an increased risk for developing alcoholic cirrhosis and HCC.[50,51] A recent meta-analysis comparing HCC patients with underlying alcoholic cirrhosis to healthy controls with the wild type CC genotype found that the CG genotype had an OR of 2.87 (95% CI: 1.61-510) for developing HCC.[50] Healthy controls were defined as patients without any evidence of ALD; data on the alcohol consumption of these participants was not reported. Patients with the GG polymorphism had a nearly 6-fold higher risk for developing HCC, with an odds ratio of 12.41 (95% CI: 6.99-22.03).[50] Salameh and colleagues[50] performed a similar analysis but changed the control group to patients with alcoholic cirrhosis. Patients with the CG and GG SNPs showed an elevated risk for developing HCC, OR 1.43 (95% CI, 0.76–2.72) and OR 2.81 (95% CI, 1.57–5.01), respectively. It should be noted that in the case of the GG polymorphism, there was a high degree of heterogeneity (I^2 = 70.38%, P =.018). Similarly, a seminal meta-analysis ascertained the risk for developing HCC among patients with the rs738409 C>G polymorphism relative to controls with alcoholic cirrhosis.[51] Consistent with other studies, an adjusted OR of 2.13 (95% CI, 1.73–2.61) was observed. Unlike the findings from other meta-analyses, this study included individual participant data (IPD) to mitigate the effects of confounders and exhibited minimal heterogeneity.

Additionally, studies have found some evidence of SNPs in other pathways that have shown an increased risk for developing HCC in the setting of alcoholic cirrhosis. These studies have explored SNPs implicated in multiple pathways, including those related to angiogenesis,[52,53] the enzymes involved in metabolizing alcohol,[54–56] myeloperoxidase,[57] and methylene tetrahydrofolate reductase.[58] However, findings from candidate gene studies, especially those studying polymorphisms involved in alcohol metabolism, are unequivocally affected by factors such as race, ethnicity, and the control group chosen.

Large-scale prospective, mechanistic, and genome-wide association studies are needed to identify, validate, and investigate the effects of SNPs on the pathogenesis of ALD and the development of HCC. Ultimately, the identification of the true underlying genetic factors can be transformational in aiding the development of targeted therapeutics as well as enhanced clinical management of at-risk patients.

Diabetes and Obesity

Multiple meta-analyses have shown that diabetes is associated with an overall 1.8-fold to 2.5-fold increased risk of developing HCC.[59–61] Although significant, these findings should be interpreted with mild caution given the heterogeneity of the studies.

Multiple studies have found that diabetes is an independent risk factor for developing HCC among patients with alcoholic cirrhosis.[9,62] In a prospective study of 478 compensated-alcoholic cirrhosis patients, diabetes had an HR of 1.6 (95% CI, 1.1–2.3; P = .029).[9] Even as a cofactor, alcohol interacts with diabetes to synergistically increase the risk for HCC.[37,63] In a population-based case-control study in Los Angeles, Yuan and colleagues[63] observed a 4.2-fold increased risk (95% CI, 2.6–5.8) among diabetics who consume more than 4 drinks per day. A hospital-based case-control study found a slightly lower, albeit still synergistic, effect among diabetic patients who consumed greater than 80 mL of alcohol per day, a 2.9-times increased risk (95% CI, 1.3–4.6).

Similarly, obesity has been linked with an increased risk for HCC among patients with alcoholic cirrhosis.[9,64] N'Kontchou and colleagues[9] found that being obese, defined as a BMI greater than or equal to 30, carried an HR of 2.9 (95% CI, 1.7–4.9; P = .0001) for developing HCC. Additionally, the investigators discovered a statistically significant interaction between BMI and diabetes in the risk for developing HCC. When analyzed together, the adjusted HR for patients with BMI greater than or equal to 30 with (n = 37) and without (n = 73) diabetes were 6.0 (95% CI, 3.7–9.7; P = .0001) and 2.1 (95% CI, 1.3–3.4; P = .002), respectively. Similar to diabetes, obesity interacts synergistically with alcohol to increase the risk for developing HCC.[65,66] A landmark prospective study of 2260 Taiwanese men from the Risk Evaluation of Viral Load Elevation and Associated Liver Disease/Cancer-Hepatitis B Virus (REVEAL-HBV) cohort found that alcohol and extreme obesity (World Health Organization definition of BMI ≥30) interact in a multiplicative, synergistic manner to increase the risk for developing HCC (adjusted HR 3.40; 95% CI, 1.24–9.34; P<.025).[65] In both of these studies, the presence or absence of concomitant NASH was not evaluated by biopsy which, if present, would play a sizable role.

SUMMARY

The linkage between compensated ALD-associated cirrhosis and HCC is best characterized as medium–high risk. The risk of developing cirrhosis and HCC increases with age and with quantity and duration of alcohol use and is exacerbated in women. Currently, the best way to reduce HCC risk is with abstinence. However, its effect is largely dependent on the severity of liver damage at the point of cessation. Some studies have shown that an elevated HCC risk may exist for decades after cessation. Furthermore, alcohol interacts with other etiologies and conditions such as viral hepatitis, hereditary hemochromatosis, diabetes, and obesity to increase the risk for developing HCC, either synergistically or additively. More studies, especially mechanistic and genome-wide association studies, are needed to definitively determine which SNPs are risk factors for the onset of ALD and its progression to HCC. Ultimately, continued progress in molecular genetics may lead to the development of targeted therapeutics for ALD, cirrhosis, and HCC which could substantially improve the management of at-risk patients.

REFERENCES

1. Kim WR, Lake JR, Smith JM, et al. OPTN/SRTR 2013 annual data report: liver. Am J Transplant 2015;15(Suppl 2):1–28.
2. El-Serag HB. Hepatocellular carcinoma. N Engl J Med 2011;365(12):1118–27.
3. Yang JD, Harmsen WS, Slettedahl SW, et al. Factors that affect risk for hepatocellular carcinoma and effects of surveillance. Clin Gastroenterol Hepatol 2011;9(7):617–23.e1.

4. World Health Organization. Global status report on alcohol and health 2014. Geneva (Switzerland): World Health Organization; 2014. Available at: http://apps.who.int/iris/bitstream/10665/112736/1/9789240692763_eng.pdf. Accessed August 14, 2015.
5. Fattovich G, Stroffolini T, Zagni I, et al. Hepatocellular carcinoma in cirrhosis: incidence and risk factors. Gastroenterology 2004;127(5 Suppl 1):S35–50.
6. Toshikuni N, Izumi A, Nishino K, et al. Comparison of outcomes between patients with alcoholic cirrhosis and those with hepatitis C virus-related cirrhosis. J Gastroenterol Hepatol 2009;24(7):1276–83.
7. Jepsen P, Ott P, Andersen PK, et al. Risk for hepatocellular carcinoma in patients with alcoholic cirrhosis: a Danish nationwide cohort study. Ann Intern Med 2012; 156(12):841–7. W295.
8. Uetake S, Yamauchi M, Itoh S, et al. Analysis of risk factors for hepatocellular carcinoma in patients with HBs antigen- and anti-HCV antibody-negative alcoholic cirrhosis: clinical significance of prior hepatitis B virus infection. Alcohol Clin Exp Res 2003;27(8 Suppl):47S–51S.
9. N'Kontchou G, Paries J, Htar MT, et al. Risk factors for hepatocellular carcinoma in patients with alcoholic or viral C cirrhosis. Clin Gastroenterol Hepatol 2006;4(8): 1062–8.
10. Mancebo A, Gonzalez-Dieguez ML, Cadahia V, et al. Annual incidence of hepatocellular carcinoma among patients with alcoholic cirrhosis and identification of risk groups. Clin Gastroenterol Hepatol 2013;11(1):95–101.
11. Ioannou GN, Splan MF, Weiss NS, et al. Incidence and predictors of hepatocellular carcinoma in patients with cirrhosis. Clin Gastroenterol Hepatol 2007;5(8): 938–45, 945.e1–4.
12. Lin CW, Lin CC, Mo LR, et al. Heavy alcohol consumption increases the incidence of hepatocellular carcinoma in hepatitis B virus-related cirrhosis. J Hepatol 2013; 58(4):730–5.
13. Simao A, Madaleno J, Silva N, et al. Plasma osteopontin is a biomarker for the severity of alcoholic liver cirrhosis, not for hepatocellular carcinoma screening. BMC Gastroenterol 2015;15:73.
14. Teli MR, Day CP, Burt AD, et al. Determinants of progression to cirrhosis or fibrosis in pure alcoholic fatty liver. Lancet 1995;346(8981):987–90.
15. Bagnardi V, Blangiardo M, La Vecchia C, et al. A meta-analysis of alcohol drinking and cancer risk. Br J Cancer 2001;85(11):1700–5.
16. Savolainen VT, Liesto K, Mannikko A, et al. Alcohol consumption and alcoholic liver disease: evidence of a threshold level of effects of ethanol. Alcohol Clin Exp Res 1993;17(5):1112–7.
17. Bellentani S, Saccoccio G, Costa G, et al. Drinking habits as cofactors of risk for alcohol induced liver damage. The Dionysos Study Group. Gut 1997;41(6): 845–50.
18. Corrao G, Bagnardi V, Zambon A, et al. Meta-analysis of alcohol intake in relation to risk of liver cirrhosis. Alcohol Alcohol 1998;33(4):381–92.
19. Becker U, Deis A, Sorensen TI, et al. Prediction of risk of liver disease by alcohol intake, sex, and age: a prospective population study. Hepatology 1996;23(5): 1025–9.
20. Donato F, Tagger A, Gelatti U, et al. Alcohol and hepatocellular carcinoma: the effect of lifetime intake and hepatitis virus infections in men and women. Am J Epidemiol 2002;155(4):323–31.
21. Rehm J, Taylor B, Mohapatra S, et al. Alcohol as a risk factor for liver cirrhosis: a systematic review and meta-analysis. Drug Alcohol Rev 2010;29(4):437–45.

22. Wacholder S, Silverman DT, McLaughlin JK, et al. Selection of controls in case-control studies. II. Types of controls. Am J Epidemiol 1992;135(9):1029–41.
23. Lu XL, Luo JY, Tao M, et al. Risk factors for alcoholic liver disease in China. World J Gastroenterol 2004;10(16):2423–6.
24. Tsukuma H, Hiyama T, Tanaka S, et al. Risk factors for hepatocellular carcinoma among patients with chronic liver disease. N Engl J Med 1993;328(25):1797–801.
25. Heckley GA, Jarl J, Asamoah BO, et al. How the risk of liver cancer changes after alcohol cessation: a review and meta-analysis of the current literature. BMC Cancer 2011;11:446.
26. Pares A, Caballeria J, Bruguera M, et al. Histological course of alcoholic hepatitis. Influence of abstinence, sex and extent of hepatic damage. J Hepatol 1986;2(1): 33–42.
27. Poynard T, Mathurin P, Lai CL, et al. A comparison of fibrosis progression in chronic liver diseases. J Hepatol 2003;38(3):257–65.
28. Baraona E, Abittan CS, Dohmen K, et al. Gender differences in pharmacokinetics of alcohol. Alcohol Clin Exp Res 2001;25(4):502–7.
29. Frezza M, di Padova C, Pozzato G, et al. High blood alcohol levels in women. The role of decreased gastric alcohol dehydrogenase activity and first-pass metabolism. N Engl J Med 1990;322(2):95–9.
30. Marshall AW, Kingstone D, Boss M, et al. Ethanol elimination in males and females: relationship to menstrual cycle and body composition. Hepatology 1983;3(5):701–6.
31. Gavaler JS. Alcohol effects on hormone levels in normal postmenopausal women and in postmenopausal women with alcohol-induced cirrhosis. Recent Dev Alcohol 1995;12:199–208.
32. Ikejima K, Enomoto N, Iimuro Y, et al. Estrogen increases sensitivity of hepatic Kupffer cells to endotoxin. Am J Physiol 1998;274(4 Pt 1):G669–76.
33. Thurman RG. Sex-related liver injury due to alcohol involves activation of Kupffer cells by endotoxin. Can J Gastroenterol 2000;14(Suppl D):129D–35D.
34. Yin M, Ikejima K, Wheeler MD, et al. Estrogen is involved in early alcohol-induced liver injury in a rat enteral feeding model. Hepatology 2000;31(1):117–23.
35. Douds AC, Cox MA, Iqbal TH, et al. Ethnic differences in cirrhosis of the liver in a British city: alcoholic cirrhosis in South Asian men. Alcohol Alcohol 2003;38(2): 148–50.
36. Cochrane R, Bal S. The drinking habits of Sikh, Hindu, Muslim and white men in the West Midlands: a community survey. Br J Addict 1990;85(6):759–69.
37. Hassan MM, Hwang LY, Hatten CJ, et al. Risk factors for hepatocellular carcinoma: synergism of alcohol with viral hepatitis and diabetes mellitus. Hepatology 2002;36(5):1206–13.
38. Chung NS, Kwon OS, Park CH, et al. A comparative cross-sectional study of the development of hepatocellular carcinoma in patients with liver cirrhosis caused by hepatitis B virus, alcohol, or combination of hepatitis b virus and alcohol. Korean J Gastroenterol 2007;49(6):369–75 [in Korean].
39. Wang LY, You SL, Lu SN, et al. Risk of hepatocellular carcinoma and habits of alcohol drinking, betel quid chewing and cigarette smoking: a cohort of 2416 HBsAg-seropositive and 9421 HBsAg-seronegative male residents in Taiwan. Cancer Causes Control 2003;14(3):241–50.
40. Gish RG, Given BD, Lai CL, et al. Chronic hepatitis B: virology, natural history, current management and a glimpse at future opportunities. Antiviral Res 2015;121: 47–58.

41. Kwon OS, Jung YK, Bae KS, et al. Anti-hepatitis B core positivity as a risk factor for hepatocellular carcinoma in alcoholic cirrhosis: a case-control study. Alcohol 2012;46(6):537–41.

42. Poynard T, Bedossa P, Opolon P. Natural history of liver fibrosis progression in patients with chronic hepatitis C. The OBSVIRC, METAVIR, CLINIVIR, and DOSVIRC groups. Lancet 1997;349(9055):825–32.

43. Wiley TE, McCarthy M, Breidi L, et al. Impact of alcohol on the histological and clinical progression of hepatitis C infection. Hepatology 1998;28(3):805–9.

44. Aizawa Y, Shibamoto Y, Takagi I, et al. Analysis of factors affecting the appearance of hepatocellular carcinoma in patients with chronic hepatitis C. A long term follow-up study after histologic diagnosis. Cancer 2000;89(1):53–9.

45. Ikeda K, Saitoh S, Koida I, et al. A multivariate analysis of risk factors for hepatocellular carcinogenesis: a prospective observation of 795 patients with viral and alcoholic cirrhosis. Hepatology 1993;18(1):47–53.

46. Tagger A, Donato F, Ribero ML, et al. Case-control study on hepatitis C virus (HCV) as a risk factor for hepatocellular carcinoma: the role of HCV genotypes and the synergism with hepatitis B virus and alcohol. Brescia HCC Study. Int J Cancer 1999;81(5):695–9.

47. Tsutsumi M, Ishizaki M, Takada A. Relative risk for the development of hepatocellular carcinoma in alcoholic patients with cirrhosis: a multiple logistic-regression coefficient analysis. Alcohol Clin Exp Res 1996;20(4):758–62.

48. Scotet V, Merour MC, Mercier AY, et al. Hereditary hemochromatosis: effect of excessive alcohol consumption on disease expression in patients homozygous for the C282Y mutation. Am J Epidemiol 2003;158(2):129–34.

49. Fletcher LM, Dixon JL, Purdie DM, et al. Excess alcohol greatly increases the prevalence of cirrhosis in hereditary hemochromatosis. Gastroenterology 2002;122(2):281–9.

50. Salameh H, Raff E, Erwin A, et al. PNPLA3 gene polymorphism is associated with predisposition to and severity of alcoholic liver disease. Am J Gastroenterol 2015;110(6):846–56.

51. Trepo E, Nahon P, Bontempi G, et al. Association between the PNPLA3 (rs738409 C>G) variant and hepatocellular carcinoma: evidence from a meta-analysis of individual participant data. Hepatology 2014;59(6):2170–7.

52. Machado MV, Cortez-Pinto H. Proangiogenic factors in the development of HCC in alcoholic cirrhosis. Clin Res Hepatol Gastroenterol 2015;39(Suppl 1):S104–8.

53. Machado MV, Janeiro A, Miltenberger-Miltenyi G, et al. Genetic polymorphisms of proangiogenic factors seem to favor hepatocellular carcinoma development in alcoholic cirrhosis. Eur J Gastroenterol Hepatol 2014;26(4):438–43.

54. Druesne-Pecollo N, Tehard B, Mallet Y, et al. Alcohol and genetic polymorphisms: effect on risk of alcohol-related cancer. Lancet Oncol 2009;10(2):173–80.

55. He L, Deng T, Luo HS. Alcohol dehydrogenase 1C (ADH1C) gene polymorphism and alcoholic liver cirrhosis risk: a meta analysis. Int J Clin Exp Med 2015;8(7):11117–24.

56. Zintzaras E, Stefanidis I, Santos M, et al. Do alcohol-metabolizing enzyme gene polymorphisms increase the risk of alcoholism and alcoholic liver disease? Hepatology 2006;43(2):352–61.

57. Nahon P, Sutton A, Rufat P, et al. Myeloperoxidase and superoxide dismutase 2 polymorphisms comodulate the risk of hepatocellular carcinoma and death in alcoholic cirrhosis. Hepatology 2009;50(5):1484–93.

58. Saffroy R, Pham P, Chiappini F, et al. The MTHFR 677C T polymorphism is associated with an increased risk of hepatocellular carcinoma in patients with alcoholic cirrhosis. Carcinogenesis 2004;25(8):1443–8.
59. El-Serag HB, Hampel H, Javadi F. The association between diabetes and hepatocellular carcinoma: a systematic review of epidemiologic evidence. Clin Gastroenterol Hepatol 2006;4(3):369–80.
60. Wang C, Wang X, Gong G, et al. Increased risk of hepatocellular carcinoma in patients with diabetes mellitus: a systematic review and meta-analysis of cohort studies. Int J Cancer 2012;130(7):1639–48.
61. Chen J, Han Y, Xu C, et al. Effect of type 2 diabetes mellitus on the risk for hepatocellular carcinoma in chronic liver diseases: a meta-analysis of cohort studies. Eur J Cancer Prev 2015;24(2):89–99.
62. Torisu Y, Ikeda K, Kobayashi M, et al. Diabetes mellitus increases the risk of hepatocarcinogenesis in patients with alcoholic cirrhosis: a preliminary report. Hepatol Res 2007;37(7):517–23.
63. Yuan JM, Govindarajan S, Arakawa K, et al. Synergism of alcohol, diabetes, and viral hepatitis on the risk of hepatocellular carcinoma in blacks and whites in the U.S. Cancer 2004;101(5):1009–17.
64. Archambeaud I, Auble H, Nahon P, et al. Risk factors for hepatocellular carcinoma in Caucasian patients with non-viral cirrhosis: the importance of prior obesity. Liver Int 2015;35(7):1872–6.
65. Loomba R, Yang HI, Su J, et al. Obesity and alcohol synergize to increase the risk of incident hepatocellular carcinoma in men. Clin Gastroenterol Hepatol 2010; 8(10):891–8, 898.e1–2.
66. Marrero JA, Fontana RJ, Fu S, et al. Alcohol, tobacco and obesity are synergistic risk factors for hepatocellular carcinoma. J Hepatol 2005;42(2):218–24.
67. Miyakawa H, Sato C, Izumi N, et al. Hepatitis C virus infection and alcoholic liver cirrhosis in Japan: its contribution to the development of hepatocellular carcinoma. Alcohol Alcohol Suppl 1993;1A:85–90.

The Effects of Alcohol on Other Chronic Liver Diseases

Christine C. Hsu, MD[a], Kris V. Kowdley, MD[b],*

KEYWORDS

- Alcohol • Nonalcoholic steatohepatitis (NASH) • Hepatitis B • Hepatitis C • Cirrhosis
- Hepatocellular carcinoma

KEY POINTS

- Alcohol often acts in synergy with other chronic liver diseases to accelerate liver injury.
- Alcohol consumption in conjunction with other chronic liver diseases can accelerate hepatic fibrosis and increase risks of cirrhosis, hepatocellular carcinoma (HCC), and liver-related mortality.
- Modest alcohol consumption has been shown to be associated with less nonalcoholic fatty liver disease (NAFLD) and nonalcoholic steatohepatitis (NASH).

Alcoholic liver disease includes a spectrum of disorders, ranging from hepatic steatosis to alcoholic hepatitis to cirrhosis. Approximately 90% of heavy drinkers (defined as >60 g of alcohol per day) have a fatty liver.[1,2] Only 30% to 35% of heavy drinkers, however, demonstrate progression to severe hepatic fibrosis and cirrhosis.[3]

The American Association for the Study of Liver Disease and European Association for the Study of the Liver define significant alcohol drinking as greater than 30 g per day in men and greater than 20 g per day in women.[4,5] The National Institute of Alcohol Abuse and Alcoholism defines binge drinking to be more than 40 g per day in women and 50 g per day in men (within 2 hours).[4]

EFFECT OF ALCOHOL ON NONALCOHOLIC FATTY LIVER DISEASE

NAFLD is increasingly recognized in the United States along with the increase in obesity and type 2 diabetes mellitus. Approximately 30% to 40% of the population in United States (80–100 million) have NAFLD.[6] NAFLD is characterized by bland steatosis, with minimal inflammation, and has a more benign course, with less than 4%

[a] Division of Gastroenterology, University of Pennsylvania, 3400 Spruce Street, Philadelphia, PA 19146, USA; [b] Swedish Liver Care Network, Swedish Medical Center, 1124 Columbia Street, Suite 600, Seattle, WA 98104, USA
* Corresponding author.
E-mail address: kris.kowdley@swedish.org

Clin Liver Dis 20 (2016) 581–594
http://dx.doi.org/10.1016/j.cld.2016.02.013
1089-3261/16/$ – see front matter © 2016 Elsevier Inc. All rights reserved.

liver.theclinics.com

progress to cirrhosis.[7] In 1980, Ludwig and colleagues[8] originally coined the term, *NASH*, to describe a liver disease that was histologically indistinguishable from alcoholic steatohepatitis but not associated with alcohol consumption. NASH is characterized histologically by hepatic steatosis, hepatocyte ballooning, lobular inflammation, and fibrosis.[9] Patients with NASH have an increased risk of advanced liver disease and 21% to 28% progress to cirrhosis.[7,10] NASH has also been identified as a cause of cryptogenic cirrhosis.[11] Therefore, the number of cases of end-stage liver disease or liver cancer due to NASH may be underestimated.

The pathogenesis of NASH remains complex; the central features are insulin resistance and metabolic disturbances that lead to increased hepatic steatosis and lipotoxicity from free fatty acids, along with oxidative stress.[7,12,13] This then leads to hepatocyte apoptosis, inflammation, activation of hepatic stellate cells, and subsequent fibrosis.[12] Risk factors for progressive NASH include factors associated with metabolic syndrome, such as increased waist circumference, hypertension, hyperlipidemia, type 2 diabetes mellitus or insulin resistance, and a family history of type 2 diabetes mellitus.[7,14–16] Human patatin-like phospholipase domain-containing 3 (PNPLA3) gene mutation has also been associated with the presence of NAFLD regardless of environmental factors and associated with more severe histopathology.[17,18]

Alcohol use has been associated with increased risks of NAFLD and fibrosis progression in NAFLD in both animal and clinical studies. In animal studies, mice that were fed a high-fat diet along with alcohol showed more evidence of inflammatory foci, hepatocyte apoptosis, increased profibrogenic gene expression, and hepatic fibrosis.[19,20] In the Dionysos Study, heavy drinkers (>30 g/d) had a 2.8-fold increased risk for hepatic steatosis, and the risk was even more pronounced (5.8-fold) for those who were obese and drank heavily (**Table 1**).[21] The synergy between obesity and alcohol consumption was further observed in the Rancho Bernardo Study where drinking greater than 3 alcoholic drinks per day and being obese increased risks of alanine aminotransferase (ALT) elevation by almost 8.9-fold (95% CI, 2.4–33.1).[22] In a cohort of 71 patients with biopsy-proved NAFLD, binge drinking was higher in patients with evidence of fibrosis progression than those without (47% vs 11%; $P = .003$). Although not statistically significant, there was a trend of increased weekly alcohol consumption in patients with evidence of fibrosis progression (38 g/wk vs 17 g/wk; $P = .061$) (**Table 1**).[23] Moreover, moderate to heavy alcohol intake (20–50 g/d and >50 g/d) was associated with increased risk of NAFLD in female patients (OR 3.35; $P = .002$), independent of body mass index (BMI), increased waist circumference, high-density lipoprotein, low-density lipoprotein, triglyceride, and fasting plasma glucose levels.[24]

In contrast, many clinical studies have also shown that light or modest alcohol consumption may be associated with lower rates of NAFLD, particularly in male patients or obese male patients.[25–28] Patients with biopsy-proved NAFLD had less NASH (OR 0.56; 95% CI 0.39–0.84, $P = .002$) and less fibrosis (OR 0.56; 95% CI, 0.41–0.78, $P = .0005$) if they were modest drinkers (<20 g/d) (**Table 1**).[27] In another study, only modest wine drinking (<10 g/d) and not modest beer or liquor drinking was associated with less NAFLD (**Table 1**).[29] In 1055 male patients with metabolic syndrome, modest drinking (20 g/d) was associated with less NAFLD and lower aspartate aminotransferase (AST), ALT, BMI, and waist circumference (**Table 1**).[25] In another Japanese cohort an inverse relationship was observed between amount of alcohol consumed per week and prevalence of fatty liver in male patients (**Table 1**).[28] The prevalence of NAFLD was 40% in male nondrinkers, and 24% in men who drank 7 drinks per week ($P<.001$). Alcohol consumption was associated with lower prevalence of fatty liver in men (OR 0.54; 95% CI, 0.56–0.68) but not in women (OR 0.80; 95% CI,

0.57–1.12; not significant). Hamaguchi and colleagues[30] showed that all forms of alcohol consumption (whether light or heavy) were protective in men, but only light and moderate drinking was protective in women (**Table 1**). However, one study (132 patients), showed that light to moderate intake to be only protective against insulin resistance but not against hepatic fibrosis or inflammation.[31] However, all the patients in this cohort underwent bariatric surgery and the majority already had advanced steatohepatitis with fibrosis.

The mechanism whereby moderate alcohol consumption may protect against NASH remains to be further elucidated. NASH patients have increased intestine permeability and endotoxemia, and regular alcohol consumption (<140 g/wk) has been associated with lower endotoxin levels and anti-endotoxin core antibodies (EndoCab) immunoglobulin G (antibody associated with host response to endotoxin).[32] Low adiponectin levels is an independent predictor of NASH and moderate alcohol consumption has been associated with higher adiponectin levels and improved insulin sensitivity.[33–36] Any alcohol consumption, however, has been associated with increased risks (hazard ratio 3.6; 95% CI, 1.5–8.3; $P = .003$) of hepatocellular carcinoma (HCC) in NASH patients.[37] Thus, the overall risks of alcohol use need to be weighed against its protective effects on NAFLD.

ALCOHOL AND HEPATITIS C

Hepatitis C is a leading cause of liver disease in United States, and National Health and Nutrition Examination Survey data from 2003 to 2010 show that 3.6 million people in the United States have positive antibodies and 2.7 million are currently infected.[38] With the addition of under-represented populations, such as prisoners, homeless or hospitalized people, and those living on Indian reservations, approximately 4.6 million people in the United States have been exposed to hepatitis C, and 3.7 million have current infection.[39] The Centers for Disease Control and the United States Preventive Services Task Force recommend hepatitis C virus (HCV) screening for patients born between 1945 and 1965.[40]

Alcoholism is often a comorbid condition in chronic hepatitis C. Hepatitis C seropositivity has been described to range from 15% to 35% of alcoholic patients.[41–43] In a study of 11,456 patients from Norway, hepatitis C prevalence was more than 7 times higher in patients with a history of alcoholism than in those without.[44]

Alcohol and hepatitis C act in synergy by increasing liver damage by means of increasing HCV viral load, oxidative stress, immune modulation, and hepatocyte toxicity.[45–47]

Alcohol can increase HCV replication in a concentration-dependent manner.[45] Severe combined immunodeficiency (SCID) mice transplanted with HCV-infected human hepatocytes demonstrate persistence of HCV infection if fed an ethanol diet as opposed to clearance in 5 weeks if fed a control diet.[48] Bukong and colleagues[49] showed that ethanol increases HCV replication by means of increased micro-RNA 122 expression. Heat shock protein 90 inhibitors decreased micro-RNA 122 expression and attenuated ethanol-induced HCV viral replication in HCV-infected hepatoma cells. This was further illustrated in another study where the addition of a micro-RNA 122 inhibitor significantly increased cyclin G1 expression and prevented ethanol-induced HCV RNA increase.[50] Alternatively, Seronello and colleagues[51] suggest that ethanol-induced HCV virus replication was related to ethanol metabolism and modulation of lipid metabolism, which was attenuated by statin therapy.

Ethanol can also exacerbate hepatitis C liver injury by increasing oxidative stress.[46,52] Ethanol administration to Huh-7 cells expressing HCV core protein

Table 1
Studies on the relationship of alcohol consumption on nonalcoholic fatty liver disease

Study	Definition of Nonalcoholic Fatty Liver Disease or Nonalcoholic Steatohepatitis	Subjects	Alcohol Consumption (g/d)	Men, Odds Ratio (CI)	Women, Odds Ratio (CI)
1. Moriya,[28] Japan, 2010	Ultrasound	4957 Men 2155 Women	Any alcohol consumption	0.54 (0.46–0.63)	0.80 (0.57–1.12)
			0–10	0.75 (0.60–0.94)	0.68 (0.44–1.05)
			10–20	0.62 (0.49–0.77)	0.85 (0.48–1.51)
			20–40	0.50 (0.41–0.61)	1.26 (0.60–2.65)
			>40	0.40 (0.32–0.49)	1.13 (0.25–5.19)
2. Hamaguchi,[30] Japan, 2012	Ultrasound	10,982 Men 7589 Women	0–20	0.69 (0.60–0.79)	0.54 (0.34–0.88)
			20–40	0.72 (0.63–0.83)	0.43 (0.21–0.88)
			>40	0.74 (0.64–0.85)	1.02 (0.44–2.35)
3. Takahashi,[24] 2015	Ultrasound	8029 Men and women	Moderate 20–50	0.90 (0.78–1.04) BMI >25 0.743	0.68 (0.395–1.15) BMI >25 0.393
			Heavy >50	0.95 (0.79–1.15) BMI >25 0.618 BMI <25 1.286	3.35 (1.56–7.13) BMI >25 6.571 BMI <25 2.21
4. Hiramine,[95] Japan 2010	Ultrasound	9886 Men	<20	0.71 (0.59–0.86)	—
			20–59	0.55 (0.45–0.67)	
			>60	0.44 (0.32–0.62)	

5. Gungi,[26] Japan, 2009	Ultrasound	5599 Men	0–20 20–40 >40	**0.82 (0.68–0.99)** — **0.75 (0.61–0.93)** 0.85 (0.67–1.09) —
6. Sogabe,[25] Japan, 2014	Ultrasound and ALT ≥31	1055 Men with metabolic syndrome	<20	**0.65 (0.47–0.91)** —
7. Dunn,[29] United States, 2008	ALT >43 Excluded viral, medication-related, alcohol hepatitis	11,754 Men and women	Modest wine <20	**0.51 (0.33–0.80)** —
8. Dunn,[27] United States, 2012	Liver biopsy	198 men 384 women	<20	Less NASH: **0.56 (0.39–0.84; P = .002)** Less fibrosis: **0.56 (0.41–0.78; P = .0005)**
9. Ekstadt,[23] Sweden, 2009	Liver biopsy	71 Men and women	Episodic binge drinking Men >60 g Women >48 g	More fibrosis: **42.15 (5.390–329.57; P<.0001)**
10. Bellentani,[21] Italy, 2000	Ultrasound	3299 Men and women	>60 g/d or lifetime of 100 kg	More NAFLD: **2.8 (1.4–7.1; P<.001)**

ORs that are statistically significant are highlighted in bold.

depleted mitochondrial glutathione stores and increased mitochondrial reactive oxygen species production, cell depolarization, and death.[52] N-acetylcysteine treatment prevented cell death and mitochondrial depolarization.[52] This was suggested to be related to the decreased O branch of Forkhead box superfamily proteins (FOXO3) transcriptional activity, which is a major transcription activator of antioxidant protein, called superoxide dismutase 2.[53] Cells infected with HCV had increased nuclear FOXO3 transcriptional activity but this was decreased with addition of alcohol.[53] Hepatitis C seems to promote nuclear translocation and activation of FOXO3; conversely, ethanol suppressed arginine methylation of FOXO3 and promoted nuclear export and degradation of FOXO3.[54]

Alcohol also leads to decreased ability of dendritic cells (antigen-presenting cells) to generate cytotoxic T-cell response to HCV viral proteins.[55] In vivo studies, ethanol did not affect cell functionality or ability to endocytose but decreased the number of splenic dendritic cells.[56] It also inhibited the costimulatory molecules on dendritic cells and decreased cytokine signaling.[56] Alcohol has been directly related to increased fas-mediated hepatocyte apoptosis in hepatitis C.[47,57] Additionally, it interferes with intracellular hepatocyte interferon (IFN)-α/β signaling and significantly enhanced a full cycle of HCV replication.[58] Alcohol inhibited STAT-1 and STAT-2, which activated the transcription of IFN-related genes.[58] More recently, it was shown that acetaldehyde (an ethanol metabolite) prevented methylation of STAT-1 genes and expression of IFN-related genes and that addition of promethylating agent attenuated its effects.[59]

Alcohol use has been associated with increased risks of cirrhosis, HCC, and liver-related mortality in hepatitis C patients. In a cohort of 2235 patients, alcohol consumption of greater than 50 g daily was associated with increased risk of cirrhosis in hepatitis C patients.[60] Additionally, past excessive use of alcohol has been associated with a 2.6-fold increased risk of developing cirrhosis (odds ratio [OR] 2.6; 95% CI, 1.9–3.5).[61] Past excessive use was defined as sustained use (>5 years [y]) of 21 and 28 glasses per week in women and men, respectively. In a cohort of HCV patients from a liver clinic, the attributable fraction of patients who ever engaged in heavy alcohol use (>50 U/wk) among patients with cirrhosis was 50%.[62] In the Chronic Hepatitis Study Cohort a history of alcohol abuse was associated with an increased risk of cirrhosis of 2.32 times (95% CI, 2.08–2.59; $P<.001$).[63] Even moderate consumption of alcohol (<40 g/d) had an increased risk of fibrosis progression after a mean average of 6.3 years.[64] Increased (5.7 g/d vs 2.6 g/d; $P = .03$) or increased frequency (34.5 drinking d/y vs 8.2 drinking d/y; $P = .006$) was also associated with an increased risk of progressive fibrosis.

Out of 8250 hospitalized chronic hepatitis C patients alcohol consumption of 4 drinks per week for at least 5 years was associated with increased risk of liver-related mortality, such as complications of decompensated cirrhosis or development of HCC (OR 1.73; 95% CI, 1.03–2.81; $P = .037$).[65] Another study also showed that the combination of heavy alcohol consumption (>80 g/d) and hepatitis C was associated with an almost 100-fold increased risk of developing HCC.[66]

By contrast, Rueger and colleagues[67] showed that significant alcohol consumption (>20 g/d $\times$ 5 y) did not contribute to the increased risk of accelerated fibrosis but that older age at the time of infection, male gender, genotype 3, and intravenous drug use as a form of infection were associated with accelerated fibrosis. Hezode and colleagues[68] showed that various degrees of moderate use is important among patients consuming less than 50 g per day. Only moderate alcohol consumption (31 g/d–50 g/d in men and 21 g/d–50 g/d in women) independently predicted risk of stage F2 to F4 fibrosis. Any alcohol consumption less than 30 g per day was not predictive. These data suggest that alcohol consumption of greater than 30 g daily among hepatitis C patients is associated with an increased risk of developing advanced fibrosis and cirrhosis. In a meta-analysis that pooled 20 studies, an increased risk of cirrhosis (2.33-fold) was associated with only heavy alcohol use of at least 210 g per week to 560 g per week (30 g/d to 80 g/d).[69]

ALCOHOL AND HEPATITIS B

Hepatitis B is the leading cause of chronic liver disease worldwide. Two billion people worldwide have been exposed to the virus and an estimated 350 million have chronic infection and are at increased risk of illness and death from liver cirrhosis and HCC.[70] Despite decreases in the prevalence of hepatitis B in certain regions of the world, the overall prevalence of hepatitis B surface antigen (HBsAg)-positive people increased from 223 million in 1990 to 240 million in 2005 worldwide.[71] Endemic areas with the highest risk are Africa and Asia.[72] Based on a study that incorporated foreign-born individuals, the prevalence of hepatitis B was estimated to be close to 2.2 million in the United States.[73]

Early epidemiologic studies showed that at least 1 hepatitis B marker was positive in 50% of the chronic alcoholic patients in an outpatient setting, which is significantly higher than a matched control population.[74] Subsequent animal studies showed that SCID mice infected with hepatitis B who are fed a chronic alcohol diet have 7-fold increased serum HBV DNA levels and HBsAg levels.[75] In contrast, another animal study showed that HBV-positive transgenic mice fed a chronic alcohol diet had lower serum HBsAg concentrations in comparison to mice fed a control diet but had increased HBsAg accumulation in their livers.[76]

Heavy alcohol use among hepatitis B patients has been associated with increased risk of developing cirrhosis, HCC, and death. The 50% probability for cirrhosis occurred at a younger age (46 y vs 75 y) in patients with chronic hepatitis B (CHB) who were heavy drinkers (>50 g/d) as opposed to those who were moderate (<50 g/d) or nondrinkers.[77] Additionally, heavy alcohol use (>350 g/wk for men and >280 g/wk for women) was associated with earlier age of death (52 y vs 64 y) in patients with CHB; 93% of the deaths were related to cirrhosis and 35% from development of HCC.[78] In a large population-based Korean study, heavy alcohol use was associated with 1.5-fold (relative risk 1.5; 95% CI, 1.2–2.0) increased risk of HCC in male patients with HBsAg positivity.[79] This risk was even more pronounced in patients with hepatitis B cirrhosis. The 10-year cumulative risk of HCC was 52.8% for CHB cirrhosis patients with heavy alcohol use (>80 g/d) versus 39.8% ($P<.001$) for those with CHB cirrhosis without alcohol use.[80]

ALCOHOL AND HEMOCHROMATOSIS

Hereditary hemochromatosis is an autosomal recessive iron overload disorder that occurs from decreased hepcidin expression and increased duodenal iron absorption.[81] Iron overload can occur in the liver, heart, skin, joints, pituitary gland, pancreas, and gonads and this can lead to cirrhosis, cardiomyopathy, arthropathy, bronze skin hyperpigmentation, diabetes mellitus, hypogonadism, and hypopituitarism.[81] The most common type of hereditary hemochromatosis is *HFE*-associated hereditary hemochromatosis.[82] Approximately 80% to 90% of patients with HFE-associated hereditary hemochromatosis have the C282Y homozygous mutation.[82]

Alcohol and iron overload also seem to have an additive synergy in increasing the risk of liver disease and fibrosis in hemochromatosis. In a cohort of 378 C282Y homozygous hemochromatosis patients, chronic alcohol use was associated with increased iron stores, transferrin-iron saturation, and higher serum liver enzymes.[83] In another cohort of 224 patients with C282Y homozygous hemochromatosis, 61% of the patients who chronically consumed greater than 60 g or more daily alcohol had evidence of advanced fibrosis or cirrhosis in contrast to only 7% of nonexcessive alcohol users.[84] In a third study with C282Y homozygous hemochromatosis patients, excess alcohol use (defined as >60 g/d in men or >40 g/d in women) was associated with a 4.25-fold increased risk (OR 4.25; 95% CI, 1.49–12.2; $P = .007$) of developing accelerated fibrosis.[85] Cirrhosis also develops at an earlier age (61 y vs 75 y of age) in hereditary hemochromatosis patients with chronic heavy alcohol consumption.[77]

ALCOHOL AND AUTOIMMUNE LIVER DISEASES

Autoimmune liver diseases include primary sclerosing cholangitis (PSC), primary biliary cirrhosis (PBC), and autoimmune hepatitis.[86] The relationship between alcohol and these various autoimmune liver diseases remains to be further elucidated.

In a small nested case-control study, alcohol consumption was associated with a 3-fold increased risk of cholangiocarcinoma development in patients with PSC (OR 2.95; 95% CI, 1.04–8.3).[87] Alcoholic liver disease alone, however, is an associated risk factor for development of intrahepatic and extrahepatic cholangiocarcinoma.[88] Thus, it remains less clear if there is an additive synergy of alcohol consumption and PSC toward increased cholangiocarcinoma.

However, alcohol consumption in PSC patients was low (9%).[89] Additionally, there was no difference in the percentage of PSC patients with regular alcohol consumption among those with significant fibrosis (transient elastography score >17.3 kPa) when compared with those without significant fibrosis (22% vs 28%; $P = .57$). Moreover, there was no correlation with alcohol consumption and transient elastography scores. The number of binge drinking occasions per year was even less for PSC patients with significant fibrosis than those without significant fibrosis (4.3 binges/y vs 14.9 binges/y).

The relationship between alcohol and autoimmune hepatitis also remains to be further elucidated. In animal studies, ethanol metabolites were shown to bind to liver cytosolic proteins and cause liver injury similar to autoimmune hepatitis.[90] However, clinically, alcohol consumption was shown to be protective, against developing autoimmune hepatitis (OR 0.43, 95% CI, 0.28–0.68; $P<.01$).[91] In PBC, chronic alcohol consumption has been associated with more progressive PBC. Men and women using greater than 30 g and 20 g per day respectively had a 4.5-fold increased risk of advanced stages of PBC (OR 4.5 95%; CI, 1.3–19.8; $P<.029$).[92] Additionally, alcohol consumption was associated with a 10-fold increased risk (OR 10.294; 95% CI, 1.11–95.68) of HCC development[93]; all PBC patients who developed HCC had cirrhosis. In a separate study from, Spain and Italy, however, alcohol consumption greater than 40 g per day was not a statistically significant factor in the development of HCC in PBC patients.[94] Further studies are needed to corroborate these findings.

SUMMARY

In most chronic liver diseases, alcohol plays a synergistic role toward increased risk of advanced fibrosis, cirrhosis, hepatic decompensation, and development of HCC. Modest or light alcohol consumption may be protective, however, against development of NAFLD and NASH. Chronic alcohol use can be associated with other malignancies; therefore, the risks of alcohol consumption must be weighed against the possible protective effects.

REFERENCES

1. Tannapfel A, Denk H, Dienes HP, et al. Histopathological diagnosis of non-alcoholic and alcoholic fatty liver disease. Virchows Arch 2011;458:511–23.
2. McCullough AJ, O'Shea RS, Dasarathy S. Diagnosis and management of alcoholic liver disease. J Dig Dis 2011;12:257–62.
3. Gao B, Bataller R. Alcoholic liver disease: pathogenesis and new therapeutic targets. Gastroenterology 2011;141:1572–85.
4. European Association for the Study of Liver. EASL clinical practical guidelines: management of alcoholic liver disease. J Hepatol 2012;57:399–420.
5. O'Shea RS, Dasarathy S, McCullough AJ, Practice Guideline Committee of the American Association for the Study of Liver Diseases, Practice Parameters Committee of the American College of Gastroenterology. Alcoholic liver disease. Hepatology 2010;51:307–28.
6. Spengler EK, Loomba R. Recommendations for diagnosis, referral for liver biopsy, and treatment of nonalcoholic fatty liver disease and nonalcoholic steatohepatitis. Mayo Clin Proc 2015;90(9):1233–46.
7. Rinella ME. Nonalcoholic fatty liver disease: a systematic review. JAMA 2015;313:2263–73.
8. Ludwig J, Viggiano TR, McGill DB, et al. Nonalcoholic steatohepatitis: Mayo Clinic experiences with a hitherto unnamed disease. Mayo Clin Proc 1980;55:434–8.
9. Kleiner DE, Brunt EM, Van Natta M, et al. Design and validation of a histological scoring system for nonalcoholic fatty liver disease. Hepatology 2005;41:1313–21.
10. Matteoni CA, Younossi ZM, Gramlich T, et al. Nonalcoholic fatty liver disease: a spectrum of clinical and pathological severity. Gastroenterology 1999;116:1413–9.
11. Caldwell SH, Lee VD, Kleiner DE, et al. NASH and cryptogenic cirrhosis: a histological analysis. Ann Hepatol 2009;8:346–52.
12. Schuppan D, Schattenberg JM. Non-alcoholic steatohepatitis: pathogenesis and novel therapeutic approaches. J Gastroenterol Hepatol 2013;28(Suppl 1):68–76.
13. Noureddin M, Rinella ME. Nonalcoholic Fatty liver disease, diabetes, obesity, and hepatocellular carcinoma. Clin Liver Dis 2015;19:361–79.
14. Kowdley KV. Advances in the diagnosis and treatment of nonalcoholic steatohepatitis. Gastroenterol Hepatol (N Y) 2014;10:184–6.
15. Loomba R, Abraham M, Unalp A, et al. Association between diabetes, family history of diabetes, and risk of nonalcoholic steatohepatitis and fibrosis. Hepatology 2012;56:943–51.
16. Dixon JB, Bhathal PS, O'Brien PE. Nonalcoholic fatty liver disease: predictors of nonalcoholic steatohepatitis and liver fibrosis in the severely obese. Gastroenterology 2001;121:91–100.
17. Romeo S, Kozlitina J, Xing C, et al. Genetic variation in PNPLA3 confers susceptibility to nonalcoholic fatty liver disease. Nat Genet 2008;40:1461–5.
18. Sookoian S, Pirola CJ. Meta-analysis of the influence of I148M variant of patatin-like phospholipase domain containing 3 gene (PNPLA3) on the susceptibility and histological severity of nonalcoholic fatty liver disease. Hepatology 2011;53:1883–94.
19. Wang Y, Seitz HK, Wang XD. Moderate alcohol consumption aggravates high-fat diet induced steatohepatitis in rats. Alcohol Clin Exp Res 2010;34:567–73.
20. Gabele E, Dostert K, Dorn C, et al. A new model of interactive effects of alcohol and high-fat diet on hepatic fibrosis. Alcohol Clin Exp Res 2011;35:1361–7.

21. Bellentani S, Saccoccio G, Masutti F, et al. Prevalence of and risk factors for hepatic steatosis in Northern Italy. Ann Intern Med 2000;132:112–7.
22. Loomba R, Bettencourt R, Barrett-Connor E. Synergistic association between alcohol intake and body mass index with serum alanine and aspartate aminotransferase levels in older adults: the Rancho Bernardo Study. Aliment Pharmacol Ther 2009;30:1137–49.
23. Ekstedt M, Franzen LE, Holmqvist M, et al. Alcohol consumption is associated with progression of hepatic fibrosis in non-alcoholic fatty liver disease. Scand J Gastroenterol 2009;44:366–74.
24. Takahashi H, Ono M, Hyogo H, et al. Biphasic effect of alcohol intake on the development of fatty liver disease. J Gastroenterol 2015;50(11):1114–23.
25. Sogabe M, Okahisa T, Taniguchi T, et al. Light alcohol consumption plays a protective role against non-alcoholic fatty liver disease in Japanese men with metabolic syndrome. Liver Int 2015;35:1707–14.
26. Gunji T, Matsuhashi N, Sato H, et al. Light and moderate alcohol consumption significantly reduces the prevalence of fatty liver in the Japanese male population. Am J Gastroenterol 2009;104:2189–95.
27. Dunn W, Sanyal AJ, Brunt EM, et al. Modest alcohol consumption is associated with decreased prevalence of steatohepatitis in patients with non-alcoholic fatty liver disease (NAFLD). J Hepatol 2012;57:384–91.
28. Moriya A, Iwasaki Y, Ohguchi S, et al. Alcohol consumption appears to protect against non-alcoholic fatty liver disease. Aliment Pharmacol Ther 2011;33: 378–88.
29. Dunn W, Xu R, Schwimmer JB. Modest wine drinking and decreased prevalence of suspected nonalcoholic fatty liver disease. Hepatology 2008;47:1947–54.
30. Hamaguchi M, Kojima T, Ohbora A, et al. Protective effect of alcohol consumption for fatty liver but not metabolic syndrome. World J Gastroenterol 2012;18:156–67.
31. Cotrim HP, Freitas LA, Alves E, et al. Effects of light-to-moderate alcohol consumption on steatosis and steatohepatitis in severely obese patients. Eur J Gastroenterol Hepatol 2009;21:969–72.
32. Wong VW, Wong GL, Chan HY, et al. Bacterial endotoxin and non-alcoholic fatty liver disease in the general population: a prospective cohort study. Aliment Pharmacol Ther 2015;42:731–40.
33. Davies MJ, Baer DJ, Judd JT, et al. Effects of moderate alcohol intake on fasting insulin and glucose concentrations and insulin sensitivity in postmenopausal women: a randomized controlled trial. JAMA 2002;287:2559–62.
34. Joosten MM, Beulens JW, Kersten S, et al. Moderate alcohol consumption increases insulin sensitivity and ADIPOQ expression in postmenopausal women: a randomised, crossover trial. Diabetologia 2008;51:1375–81.
35. Chiva-Blanch G, Urpi-Sarda M, Ros E, et al. Effects of red wine polyphenols and alcohol on glucose metabolism and the lipid profile: a randomized clinical trial. Clin Nutr 2013;32:200–6.
36. Handa P, Maliken BD, Nelson JE, et al. Reduced adiponectin signaling due to weight gain results in nonalcoholic steatohepatitis through impaired mitochondrial biogenesis. Hepatology 2014;60:133–45.
37. Ascha MS, Hanouneh IA, Lopez R, et al. The incidence and risk factors of hepatocellular carcinoma in patients with nonalcoholic steatohepatitis. Hepatology 2010;51:1972–8.
38. Denniston MM, Jiles RB, Drobeniuc J, et al. Chronic hepatitis C virus infection in the United States, National Health and Nutrition Examination Survey 2003 to 2010. Ann Intern Med 2014;160:293–300.

39. Edlin BR, Eckhardt BJ, Shu MA, et al. Towards a more accurate estimate of the prevalence of hepatitis C in the United States. Hepatology 2015;62(5):1353–63.
40. Moyer VA, Force USPST. Screening for hepatitis C virus infection in adults: U.S. Preventive Services Task Force recommendation statement. Ann Intern Med 2013;159:349–57.
41. Rosman AS, Waraich A, Galvin K, et al. Alcoholism is associated with hepatitis C but not hepatitis B in an urban population. Am J Gastroenterol 1996;91:498–505.
42. Mendenhall CL, Moritz T, Rouster S, et al. Epidemiology of hepatitis C among veterans with alcoholic liver disease. The VA Cooperative Study Group 275. Am J Gastroenterol 1993;88:1022–6.
43. Galperim B, Cheinquer H, Stein A, et al. Prevalence of hepatitis C virus in alcoholic patients: role of parenteral risk factors. Arq Gastroenterol 2006;43:81–4.
44. Dalgard O, Jeansson S, Skaug K, et al. Hepatitis C in the general adult population of Oslo: prevalence and clinical spectrum. Scand J Gastroenterol 2003;38:864–70.
45. Zhang T, Li Y, Lai JP, et al. Alcohol potentiates hepatitis C virus replicon expression. Hepatology 2003;38:57–65.
46. Perlemuter G, Letteron P, Carnot F, et al. Alcohol and hepatitis C virus core protein additively increase lipid peroxidation and synergistically trigger hepatic cytokine expression in a transgenic mouse model. J Hepatol 2003;39:1020–7.
47. Pianko S, Patella S, Sievert W. Alcohol consumption induces hepatocyte apoptosis in patients with chronic hepatitis C infection. J Gastroenterol Hepatol 2000;15:798–805.
48. Osna NA, Kharbanda KK, Sun Y, et al. Ethanol affects hepatitis C pathogenesis: humanized SCID Alb-uPA mouse model. Biochem Biophys Res Commun 2014;450:773–6.
49. Bukong TN, Hou W, Kodys K, et al. Ethanol facilitates hepatitis C virus replication via up-regulation of GW182 and heat shock protein 90 in human hepatoma cells. Hepatology 2013;57:70–80.
50. Hou W, Bukong TN, Kodys K, et al. Alcohol facilitates HCV RNA replication via up-regulation of miR-122 expression and inhibition of cyclin G1 in human hepatoma cells. Alcohol Clin Exp Res 2013;37:599–608.
51. Seronello S, Ito C, Wakita T, et al. Ethanol enhances hepatitis C virus replication through lipid metabolism and elevated NADH/NAD+. J Biol Chem 2010;285:845–54.
52. Otani K, Korenaga M, Beard MR, et al. Hepatitis C virus core protein, cytochrome P450 2E1, and alcohol produce combined mitochondrial injury and cytotoxicity in hepatoma cells. Gastroenterology 2005;128:96–107.
53. Tumurbaatar B, Tikhanovich I, Li Z, et al. Hepatitis C and alcohol exacerbate liver injury by suppression of FOXO3. Am J Pathol 2013;183:1803–14.
54. Tikhanovich I, Kuravi S, Campbell RV, et al. Regulation of FOXO3 by phosphorylation and methylation in hepatitis C virus infection and alcohol exposure. Hepatology 2014;59:58–70.
55. Encke J, Wands JR. Ethanol inhibition: the humoral and cellular immune response to hepatitis C virus NS5 protein after genetic immunization. Alcohol Clin Exp Res 2000;24:1063–9.
56. Aloman C, Gehring S, Wintermeyer P, et al. Chronic ethanol consumption impairs cellular immune responses against HCV NS5 protein due to dendritic cell dysfunction. Gastroenterology 2007;132:698–708.
57. Pianko S, Patella S, Ostapowicz G, et al. Fas-mediated hepatocyte apoptosis is increased by hepatitis C virus infection and alcohol consumption, and may be

associated with hepatic fibrosis: mechanisms of liver cell injury in chronic hepatitis C virus infection. J Viral Hepat 2001;8:406–13.

58. Ye L, Wang S, Wang X, et al. Alcohol impairs interferon signaling and enhances full cycle hepatitis C virus JFH-1 infection of human hepatocytes. Drug Alcohol Depend 2010;112:107–16.

59. Ganesan M, Zhang J, Bronich T, et al. Acetaldehyde accelerates HCV-induced Impairment of innate immunity by suppressing methylation reactions in liver cells. Am J Physiol Gastrointest Liver Physiol 2015;309(7):G566–77.

60. Poynard T, Bedossa P, Opolon P. Natural history of liver fibrosis progression in patients with chronic hepatitis C. The OBSVIRC, METAVIR, CLINIVIR, and DOSVIRC groups. Lancet 1997;349:825–32.

61. Delarocque-Astagneau E, Roudot-Thoraval F, Campese C, et al, Hepatitis C Surveillance System Steering Committee. Past excessive alcohol consumption: a major determinant of severe liver disease among newly referred hepatitis C virus infected patients in hepatology reference centers, France, 2001. Ann Epidemiol 2005;15:551–7.

62. Innes HA, Hutchinson SJ, Barclay S, et al. Quantifying the fraction of cirrhosis attributable to alcohol among chronic hepatitis C virus patients: implications for treatment cost-effectiveness. Hepatology 2013;57:451–60.

63. Gordon SC, Lamerato LE, Rupp LB, et al. Prevalence of Cirrhosis in Hepatitis C Patients in the Chronic Hepatitis Cohort Study (CHeCS): A Retrospective and Prospective Observational Study. Am J Gastroenterol 2015;110:1169–77.

64. Westin J, Lagging LM, Spak F, et al. Moderate alcohol intake increases fibrosis progression in untreated patients with hepatitis C virus infection. J Viral Hepat 2002;9:235–41.

65. Zeng QL, Feng GH, Zhang JY, et al. Risk factors for liver-related mortality in chronic hepatitis C patients: a deceased case-living control study. World J Gastroenterol 2014;20:5519–26.

66. Mueller S, Millinig G, Seitz HK. Alcoholic liver disease and hepatitis C: a frequently underestimated combination. World J Gastroenterol 2009;15:3462–71.

67. Rueger S, Bochud PY, Dufour JF, et al. Impact of common risk factors of fibrosis progression in chronic hepatitis C. Gut 2015;64:1605–15.

68. Hezode C, Lonjon I, Roudot-Thoraval F, et al. Impact of moderate alcohol consumption on histological activity and fibrosis in patients with chronic hepatitis C, and specific influence of steatosis: a prospective study. Aliment Pharmacol Ther 2003;17:1031–7.

69. Hutchinson SJ, Bird SM, Goldberg DJ. Influence of alcohol on the progression of hepatitis C virus infection: a meta-analysis. Clin Gastroenterol Hepatol 2005;3: 1150–9.

70. Lavanchy D. Hepatitis B virus epidemiology, disease burden, treatment, and current and emerging prevention and control measures. J Viral Hepat 2004;11: 97–107.

71. Ott JJ, Stevens GA, Groeger J, et al. Global epidemiology of hepatitis B virus infection: new estimates of age-specific HBsAg seroprevalence and endemicity. Vaccine 2012;30:2212–9.

72. Schweitzer A, Horn J, Mikolajczyk RT, et al. Estimations of worldwide prevalence of chronic hepatitis B virus infection: a systematic review of data published between 1965 and 2013. Lancet 2015;386(10003):1546–55.

73. Kowdley KV, Wang CC, Welch S, et al. Prevalence of chronic hepatitis B among foreign-born persons living in the United States by country of origin. Hepatology 2012;56:422–33.

74. Laskus T, Radkowski M, Lupa E, et al. Prevalence of markers of hepatitis viruses in out-patient alcoholics. J Hepatol 1992;15:174–8.
75. Larkin J, Clayton MM, Liu J, et al. Chronic ethanol consumption stimulates hepatitis B virus gene expression and replication in transgenic mice. Hepatology 2001; 34:792–7.
76. Nalpas B, Pourcel C, Feldmann G, et al. Chronic alcohol intoxication decreases the serum level of hepatitis B surface antigen in transgenic mice. J Hepatol 1992; 15:118–24.
77. Poynard T, Mathurin P, Lai CL, et al. A comparison of fibrosis progression in chronic liver diseases. J Hepatol 2003;38:257–65.
78. Marcellin P, Pequignot F, Delarocque-Astagneau E, et al. Mortality related to chronic hepatitis B and chronic hepatitis C in France: evidence for the role of HIV coinfection and alcohol consumption. J Hepatol 2008;48:200–7.
79. Jee SH, Ohrr H, Sull JW, et al. Cigarette smoking, alcohol drinking, hepatitis B, and risk for hepatocellular carcinoma in Korea. J Natl Cancer Inst 2004;96: 1851–6.
80. Lin CW, Lin CC, Mo LR, et al. Heavy alcohol consumption increases the incidence of hepatocellular carcinoma in hepatitis B virus-related cirrhosis. J Hepatol 2013; 58:730–5.
81. Kanwar P, Kowdley KV. Diagnosis and treatment of hereditary hemochromatosis: an update. Expert Rev Gastroenterol Hepatol 2013;7:517–30.
82. Kanwar P, Kowdley KV. Metal storage disorders: Wilson disease and hemochromatosis. Med Clin North Am 2014;98:87–102.
83. Scotet V, Merour MC, Mercier AY, et al. Hereditary hemochromatosis: effect of excessive alcohol consumption on disease expression in patients homozygous for the C282Y mutation. Am J Epidemiol 2003;158:129–34.
84. Fletcher LM, Dixon JL, Purdie DM, et al. Excess alcohol greatly increases the prevalence of cirrhosis in hereditary hemochromatosis. Gastroenterology 2002; 122:281–9.
85. Wood MJ, Powell LW, Dixon JL, et al. Clinical cofactors and hepatic fibrosis in hereditary hemochromatosis: the role of diabetes mellitus. Hepatology 2012;56: 904–11.
86. Washington MK. Autoimmune liver disease: overlap and outliers. Mod Pathol 2007;20(Suppl 1):S15–30.
87. Chalasani N, Baluyut A, Ismail A, et al. Cholangiocarcinoma in patients with primary sclerosing cholangitis: a multicenter case-control study. Hepatology 2000; 31:7–11.
88. Welzel TM, Graubard BI, El-Serag HB, et al. Risk factors for intrahepatic and extrahepatic cholangiocarcinoma in the United States: a population-based case-control study. Clin Gastroenterol Hepatol 2007;5:1221–8.
89. Hagstrom H, Stal P, Stokkeland K, et al. Alcohol consumption in patients with primary sclerosing cholangitis. World J Gastroenterol 2012;18:3105–11.
90. Thiele GM, Duryee MJ, Willis MS, et al. Autoimmune hepatitis induced by syngeneic liver cytosolic proteins biotransformed by alcohol metabolites. Alcohol Clin Exp Res 2010;34:2126–36.
91. Ngu JH, Gearry RB, Frampton CM, et al. Autoimmune hepatitis: the role of environmental risk factors: a population-based study. Hepatol Int 2013;7:869–75.
92. Sorrentino P, Terracciano L, D'Angelo S, et al. Oxidative stress and steatosis are cofactors of liver injury in primary biliary cirrhosis. J Gastroenterol 2010;45: 1053–62.

93. Zhang XX, Wang LF, Jin L, et al. Primary biliary cirrhosis-associated hepatocellular carcinoma in Chinese patients: incidence and risk factors. World J Gastroenterol 2015;21:3554–63.
94. Cavazza A, Caballeria L, Floreani A, et al. Incidence, risk factors, and survival of hepatocellular carcinoma in primary biliary cirrhosis: comparative analysis from two centers. Hepatology 2009;50:1162–8.
95. Hiramine Y, Imamura Y, Uto H, et al. Alcohol drinking patterns and the risk of fatty liver in Japanese men. J Gastroenterol 2011;46:519–28.

Infection and Alcoholic Liver Disease

Christine Chan, MD, Josh Levitsky, MD, MS*

KEYWORDS

- Cellular immunity • Infectious disease • Alcoholic hepatitis • Cirrhosis

KEY POINTS

- Acute and chronic alcohol use affects multiple arms of the immune system by a variety of direct and indirect mechanisms.
- Dysregulation of the immune system due to alcohol use can lead to both an immunocompromised state with an increased risk of infection and a proinflammatory state contributing to acute and chronic liver disease.
- Alcohol use can alter the clinical course and treatment of patients infected with various chronic viral and bacterial illnesses such as hepatitis B, hepatitis C, human immunodeficiency virus, and tuberculosis.
- Alcoholic hepatitis is marked by a state of immune derangement, leading to an increased risk of morbidity and mortality from infection and liver failure.

THE EFFECT OF ALCOHOL ON IMMUNE RESPONSES

The body has two broad categories of defense when challenged by pathogens: innate and adaptive immunity. The initial line of defense is carried out by the innate immune response, which consists primarily of epithelial cells and immune cells (ie, cell-mediated response) such as neutrophils, monocytes, macrophages, other antigen presenting cells, and natural-killer cells.[1] The innate immune system plays a role in activating the second line of defense, the adaptive response (T and B cells), which creates immune memory to a specific pathogen for more effective responses when encountering the same pathogen in the future.[2] The innate and adaptive immune systems are closely intertwined and interact with each other via cytokines, such as tumor necrosis factor alpha (TNF-α) and interleukin (IL), and chemokines that attract additional inflammatory cells to sites of infection.

The authors have nothing to disclose.
Division of Gastroenterology and Hepatology, Northwestern University Feinberg School of Medicine, 676 North St. Clair Street, Chicago, IL 60611, USA
* Corresponding author.
E-mail address: jlevitsk@nm.org

Clin Liver Dis 20 (2016) 595–606
http://dx.doi.org/10.1016/j.cld.2016.02.014
1089-3261/16/$ – see front matter © 2016 Elsevier Inc. All rights reserved.

liver.theclinics.com

The Effect of Alcohol on the Innate Immune System

Both animal and human research studies have shown that acute and chronic alcohol use have negative effects on structural host defense mechanisms as well as on the cell-mediated response of the innate immune system (**Fig. 1**). Complex interactions between hepatocytes and the immune system are key in the development of alcohol-induced liver damage because the liver acts a primary responder to bacteria and cell wall components released in the gut in response to alcohol ingestion.[3]

Effect on gut permeability

Epithelial cells lining the skin and mucosa of the gut and airways function as the initial physical barrier of entry for pathogens, producing the first line of defense of the innate immune system. Several studies have shown that alcohol can alter this structural barrier, leading to increased gut permeability and leakage of bacteria-derived products such as lipopolysaccharide (LPS) or endotoxins into the portal circulation. Metabolism of alcohol releases metabolites such as acetaldehyde, which impair trafficking of tight junction proteins.[4] Alcohol also alters the expression of microRNAs that lead to decreased zona occludens production, further contributing to impaired integrity of tight junctions.[5] Oxidative injury from chronic alcohol use is also noted in the gut from the overproduction of nitric oxide and formation of peroxynitrite, which can damage microtubules and lead to increased gut permeability. In mice chronically fed alcohol, reactive oxygen species (ROS) release may lead to zinc deficiency, which further exacerbates gut barrier dysfunction.[3]

These gut permeability changes allow translocation of bacteria-derived products such as LPS or endotoxin to enter the blood stream and the liver via the portal system.[6–8] These endotoxins are components of gram-negative bacteria, which have been implicated in mechanisms leading to sepsis, shock, and organ failure, particularly in alcoholic patients. Once exposed, these endotoxins activate multiple cells such as Kupffer cells, endothelial cells, and hepatocytes, creating a cascade of events and leading to proinflammatory responses.[9] Thus, it is not surprising that the severity of alcohol-induced liver injury and infection risk correlates with endotoxin levels.[10] Reduction in bacterial colonization with antibiotics or lactobacillus has been shown to prevent hepatic injury in alcohol-fed rats.[11,12]

Effect on phagocytic responses

Once activated, Kupffer cells clear bacterial antigens from the circulation via phagocytosis, and produce oxidants and cytokines. This response is exaggerated in response to larger influxes of endotoxins due to alcohol, leading to accelerated production of superoxide and TNF-α via the LPS–toll-like receptor (TLR) 4 signaling pathway. LPS binds to the coreceptor LPS-binding protein (LBP) and interacts with CD14 receptor on Kupffer cells. This binding triggers intracellular signaling, which activates transcription factors such as nuclear factor $\kappa\beta$ (NF-$\kappa\beta$), which induce proinflammatory cytokine gene expression of TNF-α and IL-1β.[3] Kupffer cells in female rats demonstrate a significantly greater response to LPS than male rats and produce higher levels of TNF-α in the setting of chronic alcohol use, suggesting a possible female predisposition to alcohol-induced liver injury that is clinically well described.[13]

Paradoxically, alcohol also leads to an immunosuppressed state by altering the production and function of monocytes, macrophages and neutrophils. This effect is reflected in a reduction of bactericidal serum activity in subjects with acute alcohol intoxication and relative granulocytopenia and is seen in 10% of chronic alcoholics. In several studies, alcohol abuse induces a state of hypoplasia in the bone marrow, leading to decreased production of new granulocytes.[14] This is further exacerbated

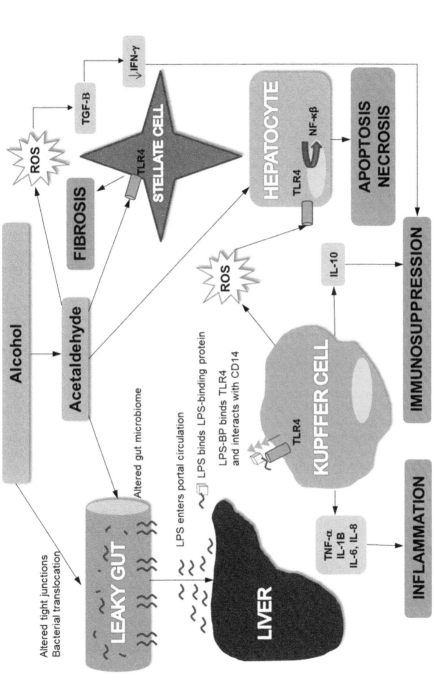

Fig. 1. Alcohol and innate immune response. Alcohol and its metabolite acetaldehyde alter tight junctions among epithelial cells, leading to increased gut permeability, allowing increased levels of lipopolysaccharide (LPS) to enter the portal circulation. LPS binds toll-like receptor (TLR) 4 and activates a cascade of cytokines and chemokines that lead to a state of both inflammation and immunosuppression. BP, binding protein; IFN, interferon; IL, inter-leukin; NF, nuclear factor; ROS, reactive oxygen species; TGF, transforming growth factor.

by malnutrition, which is common in this population.[1] During the recruitment process in the setting of infection, cell division and differentiation from precursor cells are also impaired with alcohol intoxication.[15]

Multiple steps in the delivery of these activated neutrophils to sites of infection are also affected by alcohol. Chemotaxis is reduced by circulating serum leukocyte chemotaxis inhibiting factor in the setting of alcoholic cirrhosis.[16] In addition, alcohol causes neutrophils to hyperadhere to endothelial cells, impeding diapedesis toward sites of inflammation.[17] Bactericidal capacity is reduced in neutrophils by alcohol-induced changes in membrane signaling and calcium homeostasis, leading to an over-all blunted degranulation response.[16] Alcohol abuse also affects the phagocytic function of mononuclear phagocytes, thus reducing their ability to prevent further proliferation of organisms such as mycobacteria. However, once neutrophils migrate specifically into the liver, they are actually activated by proinflammatory cytokines and induce liver damage by release of proteolytic enzymes and ROS production.[3] Thus, alcohol suppresses the neutrophils' ability to clear systemic bacterial infections but also increases their ability to induce further liver injury.

The functional quality and quantity of natural killer (NK) cells are also adversely affected by alcohol use. Cell proteins expressed by NK cells such as perforin and granzymes A and B are inhibited, leading to an impairment in the ability of these cells to destroy target cells. This mechanism is thought to play a role in increased susceptibility to viral infections and alcohol-associated tumor development.[18]

Effect on innate humoral response

Alternate pathways of alcohol-induced immunodysregulation, which do not require specific binding activity or endotoxemia, have also been noted. Suppression of interferon (IFN) secretion is noted with acute alcohol exposure, leading to increased susceptibility to bacterial infections. However, baseline levels of proinflammatory chemokines and cytokines are elevated in rats chronically fed alcohol and exacerbated by re-exposure to exogenous endotoxin.[19] Various studies have shown that in the early phase of alcohol consumption, the predominant leukocyte types are the neutrophils, after which there is a switch to higher serum levels of β-chemokines and an increased mononuclear cell infiltration, leading to more chronic liver inflammation.[19] Complement activation is suppressed in the setting of acute alcohol intoxication and increased in chronic use.[20,21]

The Effect of Alcohol on the Adaptive Immune System

Both acute and chronic alcohol use interfere with the adaptive immune response at multiple levels, including antigen presentation and proliferation of both T cells and B cells.

Effect on dendritic cells and T-cell response

Typically, dendritic cells migrate from peripheral locations to lymph nodes in the setting of infection to activate the adaptive immune response. Alcohol has been noted to affect differentiation and migration of dendritic cells to affected sites of infection.[22] Alcohol also reduces levels of costimulatory molecules (CD80 and CD86) expressed on dendritic cells, thereby impairing activation and proliferation of T cells.[2]

T helper (Th)-cell responses are adversely affected by alcohol-induced suppression of IFN-γ production, IL-2, and granulocyte-macrophage colony-stimulating factor secretion. The ability for naïve CD4 T cells to differentiate into Th1, Th17, or Th2 cells is partly mediated by IL-12 and IL-23 secretion, which is suppressed in chronic alcohol use. A shift toward favoring a Th2 response is thought to be related to these cytokine changes.[23] Impaired homeostasis in favor of Th2 cytokine release correlates with the severity of alcoholic liver disease, although the exact reason for this is not known.[1]

Chronic alcohol use is associated with reduction in number of new cytotoxic CD8+ T cells in the spleen and thymus. Existing cytotoxic T cells that express memory phenotypes, such as CD45RO, CD11b, and CD54, are, however, induced by alcohol. In one study, healthy livers in normal rats were injured by T cells derived from alcohol-fed rats.[3] Rate of progression to fibrosis and cirrhosis in patients transplanted for alcoholic liver disease who resume alcohol consumption is notably faster, suggesting a memory response by the adaptive immune system.[24]

Effect on B-cell response

Chronic alcohol use is associated with decreased B-cell response to various cytokines such as IL-2 and IL-4, reducing their ability to differentiate into plasma cells and secrete antibodies. Several studies have investigated levels of immunoglobulins in alcoholic subjects and ethanol-treated animals. Whereas some studies note elevated immunoglobulin (Ig)A, IgG, and IgM,[25] others have found significant decreases.[26] Nonetheless, the half-life of these immunoglobulins is shorter and their activity impaired with alcohol use.[1] IgE levels are notably elevated with alcohol intake, indicating activation of allergic response similar to Th2 responses.[27]

EFFECT OF ALCOHOL ON VIRAL INFECTIONS

Multiple studies have shown similarities in various mechanisms of liver injury between that of alcohol and hepatitis B virus (HBV), hepatitis C virus (HCV), and human immunodeficiency virus (HIV). LPS levels are notably elevated in patients with HIV and HCV, as they are in alcohol use.[28] Likewise, impairment of the antigen-presenting function of dendritic cells has been noted in both HIV and HCV infection with alcohol abuse.[29] Direct damage to hepatocytes via ROS production can all be independently induced by alcohol, HIV, or HCV, with a presumed additive effect. Hepatocyte death is also triggered by the induction of proinflammatory cytokine cascade, which can occur with all of these processes.

Effect on Human Immunodeficiency Virus Infection

HIV infection shares multiple common pathways with alcohol, leading to liver injury. It has been estimated that in about 17% of HIV-infected patients, death was related to end-stage liver disease, with 75% of these patients having coinfection with HCV and 48% with heavy alcohol use.[30] Heavy drinking among patients with HIV infection is thought to be twice that of the general population. Prolonged use of alcohol has also been considered a risk factor in acquiring HIV, implicating a strong social interplay between the two diseases. It has been well documented that chronic heavy alcohol use accelerates hepatic fibrosis cirrhosis in both monoinfected and coinfected HIV-positive patients.[31]

The immune modulating effects of alcohol are not only seen in the liver but can also act to alter the clinical course of HIV. Alcohol induces an increased expression of chemokine receptor (CCR5) molecules to the surfaces of monocytes, increasing HIV infection of macrophages by certain strains. Animals chronically fed alcohol have an increase in percentage of CCR5-expressing monocytes, which correlates with higher viral loads and more rapid disease progression to AIDS.[32]

Effect on Hepatitis C Virus Infection

In patients with HCV infection, alcohol affects several host factors leading to impaired immune response and higher susceptibility to hepatocyte damage. Chronic alcohol use in the setting of HCV has been associated with an increased rate of fibrosis and development of hepatocellular carcinoma, in addition to poorer response rates to treatment with IFN antiviral therapy. Furthermore, alcohol has also been noted to stimulate viral replication by potentiating HCV replicon expression, thus contributing to persistence of HCV infection.[33]

Effect on Hepatitis B Virus Infection

Similarly, HBV replication is enhanced by alcohol consumption in mouse models, with a seven-fold increase in HBV surface antigen and viral DNA levels.[34] In addition to this, alcohol activates transcription of HBV promoters via increased expression of nuclear receptors and transcription factors.[35] Alcohol use among HBV-infected patients has been associated with a significantly greater degree of piecemeal necrosis, progression to fibrosis and cirrhosis, and development of hepatocellular carcinoma.[34]

ALCOHOL USE AND PREDISPOSITION TO BACTERIAL INFECTIONS

Alcohol consumption has long been associated with systemic bacterial infections outside of its effect on liver disease and cirrhosis.[36,37] Alcohol use can alter T cells in the skin and is thus associated with increased severity of *Staphylococcus aureus* infection.[38,39] Mucosal damage caused by alcohol use has been correlated with bacterial overgrowth in the gut and there is evidence supporting chronic alcohol use and alteration in microflora toward pathogenic bacteria.[40] Decreased wound-healing capacity of epithelial cells may also contribute to a chronically impaired barrier integrity.[41]

Mechanisms of Pulmonary Injury and Increased Susceptibility to Pneumonia

Both acute and chronic alcohol abuse contributes to lung injury, with complex changes occurring in the alveolar epithelium, leading to increased risk of infection.[42] In multiple animal and cell culture models, alcohol has been found to disrupt transepithelial transport proteins and processes such as epithelial sodium channel activity (ENaC) and Na+/K+- adenosine triphosphatase (ATPase). ENaC functions to maintain healthy airway epithelium and clear extracellular fluid. The exact pathway by which alcohol upregulates ENaC activation is not entirely clear; however, alcohol-induced changes in subunit expression promote mucus stasis and inflammation, leading to a predisposition to bacterial growth and spontaneous infection.[43] Although there are discrepancies in studies investigating the exact effect of alcohol on the activity level of Na+/K+-ATPase, the overall effect of alcohol on net solute reabsorption is that of increased fluid accumulation. Like the gut, alcohol affects normal barrier function in the lung, increasing basolateral to apical leakage and bidirectional protein permeability. Multiple mechanisms have been investigated, including claudin expression leading to epithelial dysfunction and increased exposure of alveolar macrophages to pathogens.[44] Chronic alcohol abuse impairs these resident macrophages, resulting in decreased phagocytosis and increased production of ROS. In the lungs, alcohol alters nicotinamide adenine dinucleotide phosphate (NADPH) oxidase activity, which activates tissue NADPH oxidase (Nox) enzymes that produce H_2O_2 and further enhances ENaC activity. Ultimately, this leads to increased mucous production, reduction of bacterial clearance and lung injury via recruited immune cells.[45]

As a result of these effects, alcoholics are at increased risk of various pulmonary infections, most of which result from aspiration of oropharyngeal contents, including bacteria such as *Streptococcus pneumoniae* and *Klebsiella pneumoniae*. Chronic alcohol use decreases acid production in both saliva and the stomach, leading to an overall microenvironment rich in pathogenic bacterial flora. Furthermore, alcohol relaxes the lower esophageal sphincter, which contributes to the inoculation of the mouth. In the setting of alcohol intoxication, cough reflex is impaired, leading to aspiration and risk of pneumonia.[46] Studies have shown up to a seven-fold increase in mortality from bacterial pneumonia in patients reporting alcohol abuse.[47] Moreover, increased morbidity and mortality from bacterial pulmonary infections may result from alcohol's direct effect on bacterial virulence itself. In animal studies, alcohol upregulates alcohol dehydrogenase E (AdhE) and potentiates pneumolysin, increasing overall pneumococcal virulence and cytotoxicity.[48] Clinically, this process in combination with secondary injury such as septic shock hinders oxygen exchange and predisposes patients to acute respiratory distress syndrome (ARDS). Not only is there a significantly increased incidence of ARDS in those with alcohol abuse but the in-hospital mortality rate is also significantly higher.[49]

Immune Dysregulation and Bacterial Infection in Alcoholic Hepatitis

Alcoholic hepatitis (AH) is a condition of acute hepatic inflammation and injury associated with significant alcohol use. In severe presentations, one-month mortality rate can reach as high as 50%.[50] Paradoxically, AH is a complex process of both excessive systemic immune reaction and impaired immune response. Alcohol-induced derangement of the immune system via the LPS-TLRs pathway is thought to trigger a prolonged inflammatory response that leads to immune exhaustion and paralysis.[51] This process is offset by a dysregulated compensatory anti-inflammatory pathway that predisposes to infection.[52] Major causes of death in these patients include gastrointestinal bleeding, renal failure, and infection. Patients with severe AH are especially susceptible to bacterial infection and have higher rates of bacteremia, urinary tract infection, and spontaneous bacterial peritonitis.[53] Infection with *Clostridium difficile* among patients with AH is associated with higher mortality and length of stay.[54]

The optimal use of immunosuppressive therapy such as corticosteroids, pentoxifylline, and anti–TNF-α agents for AH is, therefore, controversial. Infection is typically thought to be a contraindication to corticosteroid administration. On the other hand, early therapeutic interventions may help to improve liver function and ultimately prevent further susceptibility to infection. Use of prednisolone for one month in those who are responding seems to have a beneficial effect on short-term mortality.[55] Recent studies have identified serum biomarkers differentiating systemic inflammatory response syndrome (SIRS) in the presence of infection from SIRS without infection. Levels of procalcitonin, LPS, and C-reactive protein may serve as predictors of mortality, infection risk, and treatment response in AH.[56] Early response to steroid therapy has been associated with decreased risk of infection and seems to be a more important predictor of survival.[53] Finally, although there are some data showing benefit from anti–TNF-α therapies, one trial investigating infliximab monotherapy in severe AH showed an increase risk of infection and mortality.[57]

Alcohol Use and Predisposition to Mycobacterial Infection

Although about one-third of the people in the world are infected by *Mycobacterium tuberculosis*, only 10% of those infected develop active tuberculosis (TB), usually those with impaired immune responses. Chronic alcohol use has been identified as a risk factor for both reactivation of latent disease and susceptibility to active TB. The development of active TB in chronic alcohol users is likely affected by multiple factors, including overall nutrition status, concomitant liver injury, hygienic status, and the effect of alcohol on the immune system.[58]

Alveolar macrophages are responsible for clearing more than 90% of inhaled TB mycobacteria.[59] The same mechanisms by which acute and chronic alcohol suppress overall immune function (macrophage mobilization, adherence, phagocytosis, and antigen presentation) affect alveolar macrophages and contribute to overall growth of TB. Alcohol exposure impairs the ability of alveolar macrophages to destroy TB, allowing these bacteria to survive and proliferate within them, forming tubercles in the lungs. Both CD4+ and CD8+ lymphocyte responses are altered and the ability to form granulomas to further control the spread of the disease within the host is compromised.[60] Alcohol's effect on preferentially activating a Th2 dominant immune response further hinders destruction of TB, which is predominantly overcome by Th1 activation.[61] Finally, alcohol use adversely affects the treatment course of TB because it affects the pharmacokinetics of isoniazid by decreasing its absorption and accelerating its metabolism, thereby lowering its concentration and shortening its half-life.[62]

Alcohol has been associated with extrapulmonary TB in the form of TB peritonitis (TBP). One study showed that approximately 60% of subjects with TBP have alcoholic liver disease.[63,64] Alcoholic cirrhosis has also been linked with an increased mortality rate due to TBP. Clinically, this excess mortality may be a result of late diagnosis because TBP can be challenging to diagnose in cirrhotic patients with ascites from portal hypertension. In this setting, ascitic fluid can be nondiagnostic because these patients tend to also have a low total protein and high serum-ascites albumin gradient (SAAG), with a high percentage of polymorphonuclear leukocytes similar to that of portal hypertensive ascites with spontaneous bacterial peritonitis. Acid-fast bacteria (AFB) fluid assessments and culture of ascites fluid for TB have very low sensitivity to exclude the diagnosis. Although nonspecific, LDH level greater than 90 U/L may be useful for screening for TBP before using more invasive tests such as laparoscopic peritoneal biopsy.[64] The utility of adenosine deaminase (ADA) in ascites to diagnose TBP in cirrhotic patients has been debated because ADA levels are lower in patients with cirrhosis, likely due to decreased activation of T cells in response to mycobacterial antigens. However, one study showed it was still found useful and sensitive when using a lower cut-off value.[65] Treatment with potentially hepatotoxic agents such as isoniazid and rifampin can be challenging in patients with alcoholic liver disease and cirrhosis; thus, disseminated TB in this setting often results in death from the infection or liver failure in part due to the treatment regimen.

CONTINUED RISK OF INFECTION IN PATIENTS TRANSPLANTED FOR ALCOHOLIC CIRRHOSIS

Chronic alcohol users have been noted to have a significantly higher incidence of bacterial infections following surgical procedures.[66] Likewise, patients who underwent liver transplantation for alcoholic cirrhosis have a higher incidence of bacterial gastrointestinal and pulmonary infections as well as surgical site infections during the first postoperative month compared with those transplanted for other indications. The incidence of death from sepsis is greater in patients transplanted for alcoholic cirrhosis.[67] This may be related to ongoing altered intestinal permeability that may not fully reverse until several weeks following transplantation. Although the rates of infection are higher among these patients, the rates of acute and chronic rejection are notably lower.[68] These findings suggest an overall reduced immune responsiveness to donor alloantigens, as well as bacterial pathogens in the early postoperative period. Another explanation for these findings may be an abnormal neuroendocrine-immune axis and an altered stress response leading to increased infection rates in the postoperative period.[69] The mechanism and duration of this prolonged state of immune suppression despite abstinence or full remission from alcohol is not yet known; certainly, delayed improvement in postoperative nutritional status plays a role.

SUMMARY

Alcohol is recognized as an important immunomodulator with a significant effect on multiple arms of the immune system, resulting in increased susceptibility and severity of infections that contribute to morbidity and mortality. The diverse effects of alcohol are seen in both acute and chronic use of alcohol, impairing structural host defense mechanisms that affect the course of chronic viral infections and predispose patients to bacterial and mycobacterial infections. Although alcohol acts as an immune suppressing agent, it has also been found to activate a proinflammatory response which may directly contribute to the pathogenesis of alcoholic liver disease.

REFERENCES

1. Chiapelli F. Alcohol and immune function. In: Gershwin ME, editor. Nutrition and immunology: principles and practice. Totowa (NJ): Humana Press; 2000. p. 261–74.
2. Molina PE, Happel KI, Zhang P, et al. Focus on: alcohol and the immune system. Alcohol Res Health 2010;33(1–2):97–108.
3. Duddempudi AT. Immunology in alcoholic liver disease. Clin Liver Dis 2012;16(4): 687–98.
4. Atkinson KJ, Rao RK. Role of protein tyrosine phosphorylation in acetaldehyde-induced disruption of epithelial tight junctions. Am J Physiol Gastrointest Liver Physiol 2001;280(6):G1280–8.
5. Tang Y, Banan A, Forsyth CB, et al. Effect of alcohol on miR-212 expression in intestinal epithelial cells and its potential role in alcoholic liver disease. Alcohol Clin Exp Res 2008;32(2):355–64.
6. Keshavarzian A, Holmes EW, Patel M, et al. Leaky gut in alcoholic cirrhosis: a possible mechanism for alcohol-induced liver damage. Am J Gastroenterol 1999;94(1):200–7.
7. Rao R. Endotoxemia and gut barrier dysfunction in alcoholic liver disease. Hepatology 2009;50(2):638–44.
8. Voican CS, Perlemuter G, Naveau S. Mechanisms of the inflammatory reaction implicated in alcoholic hepatitis: 2011 update. Clin Res Hepatol Gastroenterol 2011;35(6–7):465–74.
9. Fukui H, Brauner B, Bode JC, et al. Plasma endotoxin concentrations in patients with alcoholic and non-alcoholic liver disease: reevaluation with an improved chromogenic assay. J Hepatol 1991;12(2):162–9.
10. Nanji AA, Khettry U, Sadrzadeh SM, et al. Severity of liver injury in experimental alcoholic liver disease. Correlation with plasma endotoxin, prostaglandin E2, leukotriene B4, and thromboxane B2. Am J Pathol 1993;142(2):367–73.
11. Adachi Y, Moore LE, Bradford BU, et al. Antibiotics prevent liver injury in rats following long-term exposure to ethanol. Gastroenterology 1995;108(1):218–24.
12. Nanji AA, Khettry U, Sadrzadeh SM. Lactobacillus feeding reduces endotoxemia and severity of experimental alcoholic liver (disease). Proc Soc Exp Biol Med 1994;205(3):243–7.
13. Yin M, Ikejima K, Wheeler MD, et al. Estrogen is involved in early alcohol-induced liver injury in a rat enteral feeding model. Hepatology 2000;31(1):117–23.
14. Nakao S, Harada M, Kondo K, et al. Reversible bone marrow hypoplasia induced by alcohol. Am J Hematol 1991;37(2):120–3.

15. Zhang P, Welsh DA, Siggins RW 2nd, et al. Acute alcohol intoxication inhibits the lineage- c-kit+ Sca-1+ cell response to Escherichia coli bacteremia. J Immunol 2009;182(3):1568–76.

16. Jareo PW, Preheim LC, Gentry MJ. Ethanol ingestion impairs neutrophil bactericidal mechanisms against *Streptococcus pneumoniae*. Alcohol Clin Exp Res 1996;20(9):1646–52.

17. MacGregor RR, Safford M, Shalit M. Effect of ethanol on functions required for the delivery of neutrophils to sites of inflammation. J Infect Dis 1988;157(4):682–9.

18. Pan HN, Sun R, Jaruga B, et al. Chronic ethanol consumption inhibits hepatic natural killer cell activity and accelerates murine cytomegalovirus-induced hepatitis. Alcohol Clin Exp Res 2006;30(9):1615–23.

19. Bautista AP. Impact of alcohol on the ability of Kupffer cells to produce chemokines and its role in alcoholic liver disease. J Gastroenterol Hepatol 2000;15(4): 349–56.

20. Bykov I, Junnikkala S, Pekna M, et al. Effect of chronic ethanol consumption on the expression of complement components and acute-phase proteins in liver. Clin Immunol 2007;124(2):213–20.

21. Roychowdhury S, McMullen MR, Pritchard MT, et al. An early complement-dependent and TLR-4-independent phase in the pathogenesis of ethanol-induced liver injury in mice. Hepatology 2009;49(4):1326–34.

22. Ness KJ, Fan J, Wilke WW, et al. Chronic ethanol consumption decreases murine Langerhans cell numbers and delays migration of Langerhans cells as well as dermal dendritic cells. Alcohol Clin Exp Res 2008;32(4):657–68.

23. Heinz R, Waltenbaugh C. Ethanol consumption modifies dendritic cell antigen presentation in mice. Alcohol Clin Exp Res 2007;31(10):1759–71.

24. Bonet H, Manez R, Kramer D, et al. Liver transplantation for alcoholic liver disease: survival of patients transplanted with alcoholic hepatitis plus cirrhosis as compared with those with cirrhosis alone. Alcohol Clin Exp Res 1993;17(5): 1102–6.

25. Alexander GJ, Nouri-Aria KT, Eddleston AL, et al. Contrasting relations between suppressor-cell function and suppressor-cell number in chronic liver disease. Lancet 1983;1(8337):1291–3.

26. Lopez MC, Huang DS, Borgs P, et al. Modification of lymphocyte subsets in the intestinal-associated immune system and thymus by chronic ethanol consumption. Alcohol Clin Exp Res 1994;18(1):8–11.

27. Gonzalez-Quintela A, Vidal C, Gude F. Alcohol, IgE and allergy. Addict Biol 2004; 9(3–4):195–204.

28. Douek D. HIV disease progression: immune activation, microbes, and a leaky gut. Top HIV Med 2007;15(4):114–7.

29. Dolganiuc A, Kodys K, Kopasz A, et al. Additive inhibition of dendritic cell allostimulatory capacity by alcohol and hepatitis C is not restored by DC maturation and involves abnormal IL-10 and IL-2 induction. Alcohol Clin Exp Res 2003; 27(6):1023–31.

30. Salmon-Ceron D, Rosenthal E, Lewden C, et al. Emerging role of hepatocellular carcinoma among liver-related causes of deaths in HIV-infected patients: The French national Mortalité 2005 study. J Hepatol 2009;50(4):736–45.

31. Szabo G, Zakhari S. Mechanisms of alcohol-mediated hepatotoxicity in human-immunodeficiency-virus-infected patients. World J Gastroenterol 2011;17(20): 2500–6.

32. Bagby GJ, Zhang P, Purcell JE, et al. Chronic binge ethanol consumption accelerates progression of simian immunodeficiency virus disease. Alcohol Clin Exp Res 2006;30(10):1781–90.

33. Zhang T, Li Y, Lai JP, et al. Alcohol potentiates hepatitis C virus replicon expression. Hepatology 2003;38(1):57–65.

34. Larkin J, Clayton MM, Liu J, et al. Chronic ethanol consumption stimulates hepatitis B virus gene expression and replication in transgenic mice. Hepatology 2001; 34(4 Pt 1):792–7.

35. Min BY, Kim NY, Jang ES, et al. Ethanol potentiates hepatitis B virus replication through oxidative stress-dependent and -independent transcriptional activation. Biochem Biophys Res Commun 2013;431(1):92–7.

36. Nolan JP. Alcohol as a factor in the illness of university service patients. Am J Med Sci 1965;249:135–42.

37. Aguado Garcia JM, Fernandez Guerrero ML, Diaz Curiel M, et al. Bacteremic pneumonias caused by gram-negative aerobic bacilli in the adult. Apropos of 35 cases. Rev Clin Esp 1984;174(3–4):85–9 [in Spanish].

38. Parlet CP, Waldschmidt TJ, Schlueter AJ. Chronic ethanol feeding induces subset loss and hyporesponsiveness in skin T cells. Alcohol Clin Exp Res 2014;38(5): 1356–64.

39. Parlet CP, Kavanaugh JS, Horswill AR, et al. Chronic ethanol feeding increases the severity of *Staphylococcus aureus* skin infections by altering local host defenses. J Leukoc Biol 2015;97(4):769–78.

40. Bode JC, Bode C, Heidelbach R, et al. Jejunal microflora in patients with chronic alcohol abuse. Hepatogastroenterology 1984;31(1):30–4.

41. Shaw TJ, Martin P. Wound repair at a glance. J Cell Sci 2009;122(Pt 18):3209–13.

42. Downs CA, Trac D, Brewer EM, et al. Chronic alcohol ingestion changes the landscape of the alveolar epithelium. Biomed Res Int 2013;2013:470217.

43. Livraghi-Butrico A, Kelly EJ, Klem ER, et al. Mucus clearance, MyD88-dependent and MyD88-independent immunity modulate lung susceptibility to spontaneous bacterial infection and inflammation. Mucosal Immunol 2012;5(4):397–408.

44. Fernandez AL, Koval M, Fan X, et al. Chronic alcohol ingestion alters claudin expression in the alveolar epithelium of rats. Alcohol 2007;41(5):371–9.

45. Yeligar SM, Harris FL, Hart CM, et al. Ethanol induces oxidative stress in alveolar macrophages via upregulation of NADPH oxidases. J Immunol 2012;188(8): 3648–57.

46. Zhang P, Bagby GJ, Happel KI, et al. Alcohol abuse, immunosuppression, and pulmonary infection. Curr Drug Abuse Rev 2008;1(1):56–67.

47. Schmidt W, De Lint J. Causes of death of alcoholics. Q J Stud Alcohol 1972;33(1): 171–85.

48. Luong TT, Kim EH, Bak JP, et al. Ethanol-induced alcohol dehydrogenase E (AdhE) potentiates pneumolysin in *Streptococcus pneumoniae*. Infect Immun 2015;83(1):108–19.

49. Berkowitz DM, Danai PA, Eaton S, et al. Alcohol abuse enhances pulmonary edema in acute respiratory distress syndrome. Alcohol Clin Exp Res 2009; 33(10):1690–6.

50. Yu CH, Xu CF, Ye H, et al. Early mortality of alcoholic hepatitis: a review of data from placebo-controlled clinical trials. World J Gastroenterol 2010;16(19):2435–9.

51. Bataller R, Mandrekar P. Identifying molecular targets to improve immune function in alcoholic hepatitis. Gastroenterology 2015;148(3):498–501.

52. Chirapongsathorn S, Kamath PS, Shah V. Alcoholic hepatitis: can we outwit the Grim Reaper? Hepatology 2015;62(3):671–3.

53. Louvet A, Wartel F, Castel H, et al. Infection in patients with severe alcoholic hepatitis treated with steroids: early response to therapy is the key factor. Gastroenterology 2009;137(2):541–8.
54. Sundaram V, May FP, Manne V, et al. Effects of *Clostridium difficile* infection in patients with alcoholic hepatitis. Clin Gastroenterol Hepatol 2014;12(10): 1745–52.e2.
55. Thursz MR, Forrest EH, Ryder S, STOPAH Investigators. Prednisolone or pentoxifylline for alcoholic hepatitis. N Engl J Med 2015;373(3):282–3.
56. Michelena J, Altamirano J, Abraldes JG, et al. Systemic inflammatory response and serum lipopolysaccharide levels predict multiple organ failure and death in alcoholic hepatitis. Hepatology 2015;62(3):762–72.
57. Sharma P, Kumar A, Sharma BC, et al. Infliximab monotherapy for severe alcoholic hepatitis and predictors of survival: an open label trial. J Hepatol 2009; 50(3):584–91.
58. Rehm J, Samokhvalov AV, Neuman MG, et al. The association between alcohol use, alcohol use disorders and tuberculosis (TB). A systematic review. BMC Public Health 2009;9:450.
59. Dannenberg AM Jr. Immune mechanisms in the pathogenesis of pulmonary tuberculosis. Rev Infect Dis 1989;11(Suppl 2):S369–78.
60. Mason CM, Dobard E, Zhang P, et al. Alcohol exacerbates murine pulmonary tuberculosis. Infect Immun 2004;72(5):2556–63.
61. Gamble L, Mason CM, Nelson S. The effects of alcohol on immunity and bacterial infection in the lung. Med Mal Infect 2006;36(2):72–7.
62. Koriakin VA, Sokolova GB, Grinchar NA, et al. Pharmacokinetics of isoniazid in patients with pulmonary tuberculosis and alcoholism. Probl Tuberk 1986;(12): 43–6 [in Russian].
63. Chow KM, Chow VC, Hung LC, et al. Tuberculous peritonitis-associated mortality is high among patients waiting for the results of mycobacterial cultures of ascitic fluid samples. Clin Infect Dis 2002;35(4):409–13.
64. Shakil AO, Korula J, Kanel GC, et al. Diagnostic features of tuberculous peritonitis in the absence and presence of chronic liver disease: a case control study. Am J Med 1996;100(2):179–85.
65. Liao YJ, Wu CY, Lee SW, et al. Adenosine deaminase activity in tuberculous peritonitis among patients with underlying liver cirrhosis. World J Gastroenterol 2012; 18(37):5260–5.
66. Tonnesen H, Petersen KR, Hojgaard L, et al. Postoperative morbidity among symptom-free alcohol misusers. Lancet 1992;340(8815):334–7.
67. Farges O, Saliba F, Farhamant H, et al. Incidence of rejection and infection after liver transplantation as a function of the primary disease: possible influence of alcohol and polyclonal immunoglobulins. Hepatology 1996;23(2):240–8.
68. Platz KP, Mueller AR, Spree E, et al. Liver transplantation for alcoholic cirrhosis. Transpl Int 2000;13(Suppl 1):S127–30.
69. Eggers V, Pascher A, Althoff H, et al. Immune reactivity is more suppressed in patients with alcoholic liver disease than in patients with virus-induced cirrhosis after CRH stimulation. Alcohol Clin Exp Res 2006;30(1):140–9.

Moving?

Make sure your subscription moves with you!

To notify us of your new address, find your **Clinics Account Number** (located on your mailing label above your name), and contact customer service at:

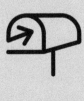

Email: journalscustomerservice-usa@elsevier.com

800-654-2452 (subscribers in the U.S. & Canada)
314-447-8871 (subscribers outside of the U.S. & Canada)

Fax number: 314-447-8029

Elsevier Health Sciences Division
Subscription Customer Service
3251 Riverport Lane
Maryland Heights, MO 63043

*To ensure uninterrupted delivery of your subscription, please notify us at least 4 weeks in advance of move.

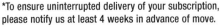

Printed and bound by CPI Group (UK) Ltd, Croydon, CR0 4YY

03/10/2024

01040394-0019